THE METABOLIC
SYNDROME
PROGRAM

THE METABOLIC SYNDROME PROGRAM

How to Lose Weight, Beat Heart Disease, Stop Insulin Resistance and More

KARLENE KARST, RD

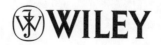

WILEY

John Wiley & Sons Canada, Ltd.

Library and Archives Canada Cataloguing in Publication Data

Karst, Karlene
    The metabolic syndrome program : how to lose weight, beat heart disease, stop insulin resistance and more / Karlene Karst.

Includes index.
ISBN-13 978-0-470-83826-6
ISBN-10 0-470-83826-4

1. Insulin resistance—Nutritional aspects—Popular works.   I. Title.
RC662.4.K37 2006   616.3'998   C2006-900973-2

Production Credits:
Cover design: Mike Chan
Interior text design: Adrian So
Printer: Transcontinental

John Wiley & Sons Canada, Ltd.
6045 Freemont Blvd.
Mississauga, Ontario
L5R 4J3

Printed in Canada
1 2 3 4 5 TRANS 10 09 08 07 06

CONTENTS

ACKNOWLEDGEMENTS

There are numerous people and influences in my life that need to be acknowledged for the success of my career and the development of this book. Most importantly, none of this would have happened without my steadfast faith in God—through Him all is possible. To my dad, who passed away 11 years ago from cancer, your memory continues to motivate and inspire me. To my family, who are my biggest fans, thank you for your continued support. To Gaetano, my husband to be, you are my rock—you have taught me so much, thank you for loving me and encouraging me to be the best person and nutritionist I can be. The greatest blessing is having a partner who shares so many of the same passions in life.

A special thank you to Nature's Way for supporting me and giving me the honor of representing your company and brand in the health and nutrition industry. It is a pleasure to have formed this relationship with such a high-quality, respectable brand.

For those in my professional life who believed in me from a very young age, especially Dean Yachison, Marc Vaugeois, Jason Mitchell, Jan Summerfeldt, and Dr. Rakesh Kapoor, I will never forget the support, opportunities and teaching you have given me.

To Joan Whitman and Valerie Ahwee for your literary expertise and the countless hours spent in making this book a success.

A book on metabolic syndrome would not be possible without the researchers and scientists in this field, especially Dr. Gerald Reaven—thank you for sharing your knowledge and expertise.

PART I

THE DAISY EXPLAINED

Chapter 1

METABOLIC SYNDROME:
A Weighty Issue

Alex Mariner, 48, has known for years that he needs to lose weight and figured he was in for another lecture when he went to see his doctor for his annual checkup. He wasn't expecting to hear that he had some strange-sounding syndrome. Alex has always been worried about developing type 2 diabetes because it runs in the family, but he never expected the doctor would tell him that he had metabolic syndrome.

Metabolic what? Alex has joined the growing number of people who have metabolic syndrome, a precursor to diabetes, a diagnosis that is becoming increasingly common, primarily because of the obesity epidemic.

An estimated 25% of the U.S. population is said to have metabolic syndrome—a mere 70 million adults age 20 and older—and the rate approaches 50% among the elderly. Mexican Americans and African-American women appear to be especially prone. Yet I would bet that most of you reading this book have never even heard about it. Why is this? There is no logical explanation for the lack of public education on the pernicious health effects of metabolic syndrome, formerly known as Syndrome X. However, it takes a while for new concepts, such as "Syndrome X," first described by endocrinologist Dr. Gerald Reaven in 1988, to become "mainstream" among the modern medical community. Early responses from the medical community to Dr. Reaven's definition were not overly positive, there are still skeptics, and experts who disagree about how dangerous it is and how intensively it should be treated. But many experts feel the metabolic syndrome approach is very useful. It has crystallized thinking about how fat causes illness, motivating people to lose weight and exercise, and prompting doctors to identify and treat people sooner.

Dr. Reaven paved the way for further research. The underlying root cause of metabolic syndrome is insulin resistance, which leads to increased cardiovascular disease and precedes type 2 diabetes. Dr. Reaven proposed that there is a metabolic defect that causes the cells' resistance to insulin. The metabolic defect is caused by a combination of heredity and lifestyle factors. In other words, insulin is present, but it does not do its job properly. This resistance to insulin sets the stage for obesity, high blood cholesterol, and hypertension.

Figure 1.1: Metabolic Syndrome

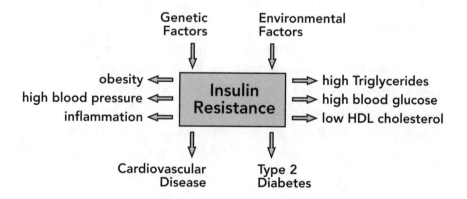

The time has come to take action. Doctors around the globe are paying attention to metabolic syndrome, which has emerged as the primary culprit of type 2 diabetes and cardiovascular disease. Soon, metabolic syndrome will overtake cigarette smoking as the number-one risk factor for heart disease among the U.S. population. With rates of diabetes expected to reach the three hundred million mark in the next two decades, and with cardiovascular disease still ranking as the number one killer in North America, metabolic syndrome has gone from being relatively unheard of to a worldwide emergency.

METABOLIC SYNDROME: THE CONCEPT

A syndrome is a collection of symptoms that make someone prone to disease. Dr. Reaven's definition of Syndrome X focused on the cluster of symptoms, in which he included insulin resistance and glucose intolerance (poor blood sugar control), obesity (although not strongly emphasized), blood-fat abnormalities (high levels of cholesterol and triglycerides), and high blood pressure. He described syndrome X as a condition triggered by an inability to respond properly to insulin, which controls blood sugar levels. He realized that instead of regarding each of the risk factors for diabetes and heart disease as separate entities, they should be viewed as connected to one another.

Clustering the components of metabolic syndrome has advantages over analyzing each of the components individually. Each factor by itself may not be highly dangerous, but together they appear to sharply boost the danger of major health problems, notably heart disease and diabetes. The risk for having coronary heart disease (CHD) is significantly greater in cases with the metabolic syndrome compared to the risk associated with each component alone. This is true in those people who have impaired glucose tolerance (prediabetic) and in patients with type 2 diabetes. Compared with non-insulin-resistant people, those with higher levels of insulin have twice as much chance of developing hypertension, three times as much chance of developing the abnormal cholesterol patterns, and five times greater chance of developing diabetes. All these are risk factors for CHD, doubling your risk of developing cardiovascular disease, with heart attack being the ultimate result if the risk factors are left untreated.

PREDIABETES AND TYPE 2 DIABETES: WHEN ONE BECOMES THE OTHER

You may have heard the term "prediabetes," which is an important concept to understand when discussing metabolic syndrome and diabetes. Prediabetes, which used to be called "impaired fasting glucose," is a precursor or intermediate stage in the natural development of diabetes. If you have blood glucose levels higher than what is considered normal but below what is considered the level for a diagnosis of diabetes, you have prediabetes. It is like the warning light in your car that comes on telling you how many miles you have to go before you run out of gas. It means that something needs to be done (you have to get gas) or you will be in trouble. Prediabetes is the same thing. It signals danger that could potentially lead to type 2 diabetes unless treated.

The diagnosis of prediabetes is based on impaired fasting glucose (IFG), which measures how much sugar/glucose is in the blood, or impaired glucose tolerance (IGT) tests. If you have IFG or IGT, you are at risk of developing type 2 diabetes. To determine if you have IFG or IGT, your doctor will have to do a fasting (no eating for 8 hours) plasma glucose (FPG) test and a 2-hour plasma glucose test (after the delivery of a 75 gram glucose drink). If your FPG is between 6.1 and 6.9 mmol/L (10 mg/dL and 124 mg/dL) and your 2-hour oral glucose is less than 7.8 mmol/L (140 mg/dL), you have impaired fasting glucose, or prediabetes. If your fasting plasma glucose is less than 6.1 mmol/L (110 mg/dL) and your 2-hour oral glucose test is 7.8 to 11.0 mmol/L (140 mg/dL and 198 mg/dL), you have impaired glucose tolerance.

The risk of developing diabetes was found to be approximately 3.6 to 3.8 percent per year in patients with IGT. Elevated fasting glucose levels, elevated 2-hour post oral glucose test, and a body mass index greater than 27 kg per m2 were associated with the development of diabetes in these patients.

Compared with people who have normal blood glucose levels, patients with IGT are at a substantially greater risk of developing cardiovascular disease.

Table 1.1: Glucose Levels for Diagnosis of IFG, IGT, and Diabetes

	Fasting Plasma Glucose (mmol/L)		2-hour Plasma Glucose after the 75 gram Oral Glucose Tolerance Test (OGTT) (mmol/L)
IFG	6.1– 6.9 (110-124 mg/dL)		N/A
IFG (isolated)	6.1– 6.9 (110-124mg/dL)	And	<7.8 (140 mg/dL)
IGT (isolated)	<6.1 (110mg/dL)	And	7.8–11.0 (140–198 mg/dL)
IFG and IGT	6.1– 6.9 (110 mg/dL)	And	7.8–11.0 (140–198 mg/dL)
Type 2 Diabetes	>/-7.0 (126 mg/dL)	Or	>/-11.1 (200 mg/dL)

Source: Adapted from the Canadian Diabetes Association

If you have higher than normal blood glucose levels, there are still opportunities to prevent or delay type 2 diabetes. Maintaining a healthy weight, participating in regular activity, and making healthy food choices can help prevent or delay the development of type 2 diabetes. (For further information see Chapter 7.)

When insulin resistance develops, the beta cells of the pancreas try to compensate by making more insulin. This helps keep blood glucose levels relatively normal, but eventually the beta cells become exhausted and cannot produce enough insulin to overcome insulin resistance. This is when impaired glucose tolerance develops in which blood glucose levels are higher than normal, but not as high as those in diabetes. Left untreated, this condition frequently progresses to full-blown type 2 diabetes.

Figure 1.2: The Progression of Diabetes

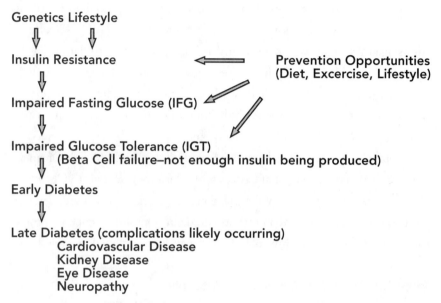

While people with isolated IFG or isolated IGT do not have the diabetes-associated risk for diseases of the small blood vessels, like eye and kidney disease, they have a higher risk for the development of diabetes and cardiovascular disease. IGT is more strongly associated with cardiovascular disease outcomes. Those who have both IFG and IGT are at a higher risk for diabetes as well as cardiovascular disease. Lifestyle interventions, including diet, exercise, and weight loss, have been highly effective in delaying or preventing the onset of diabetes in people with IGT.

A GROWING EPIDEMIC

The prevalence of metabolic syndrome will increase as the population continues to age and become more obese. Some experts predict that at least half of persons older than 60 would meet the criteria for this syndrome. Rates of metabolic syndrome also differ across ethnic groups, according to the Findings from the Third National Health and Nutrition Examination Survey. The highest overall prevalence has been found in Mexican Americans (31.9%)

and the lowest among whites (23.8%), African-Americans (21.6%), and people reporting "other" race or ethnicity (20.3%). Obesity and diabetes trends seem to mirror metabolic syndrome trends. From 1999 to 2000, 64% of U.S. adults aged 20 to 74 were overweight or obese, according to data from the Department of Health and Human Services. One study done in the United States showed that 83% of diabetics had metabolic syndrome before they were diagnosed with diabetes. A study done in Canada showed that 51% of patients with CHD had metabolic syndrome.

Metabolic syndrome has been recognized by the World Health Organization (WHO) and the National Cholesterol Education Program (NCEP), and although their definitions vary slightly, there are overlapping features between the two. They have created an operational definition of metabolic syndrome: the co-occurrence of any three of the abnormalities mentioned in Table 1.2.

Table 1.2: Diagnostic Criteria for Metabolic Syndrome According to the WHO and the NCEP ATP III

Component	Modified WHO Diagnostic Criteria (insulin resistance* plus two of the following)	NCEP ATP III Diagnostic Criteria (three of the following)
Abdominal/central obesity	Waist to hip ratio: >0.90 (men), >0.85 (women), or BMI >30 kg/m2	Waist circumference: >102 cm (40 in) in men, >88 cm (35 in) in women
Hypertriglyceridemia	≥150 mg per dl (1.7 mmol per L)	≥150 mg per dL
Low HDL Cholesterol	<35 mg per dL (0.9 mmol per L) for men, <39 mg per dL (<1.1 mmol per L) for women	<40 mg per dL (<1.036 mmol per L) for men, <50 mg per dL (1.295 mmol per L) for women
High Blood Pressure	≥140/90 mm Hg or documented use of antihypertensive therapy	≥130/85 mm Hg or documented use of antihypertensive therapy

Insulin Resistance	Fasting plasma glucose ≥7.0 mmol/l or hyperin-sulinemia (upper quartile of the non-diabetic population)	Fasting plasma glucose ≥110 mg per dL (≥6.1 mmol per L)†

WHO = World Health Organization; ATP = Adult Treatment Panel; BMI = Body Mass Index; HDL = High-density Lipoprotein

* Insulin resistance is identified by type 2 diabetes mellitus or impaired fasting glucose

† The American Diabetes Association recently has suggested lowering this threshold to 100.

Adapted from National Institute of Health: Third Report of the National Cholesterol Education Program Expert Panel on Detection, Evaluation, and Treatment of High Blood Cholesterol in Adults (Adult Treatment Panel III). Executive Summary. Bethesda, MD. World Health Organization. Definition, diagnosis and classification of diabetes mellitus. Report of a WHO consultation. Geneva: World Health Organization; 1999.

METABOLIC SYNDROME REDEFINED

Metabolic syndrome can be a difficult concept to understand. In the past, scientists like Dr. Reaven and other medical professionals have used the letter X to symbolize syndrome X or metabolic syndrome. The X represents the multidimensional components of syndrome X that account for cardiovascular disease risks. Each corner of the X represents a risk factor. The X also stands for something that is yet to be defined. With further research in large populations, the concept of metabolic syndrome has been refined. Syndrome X is now understood by the medical community, reflecting the name change to metabolic syndrome.

Figure 1.3: Syndrome X

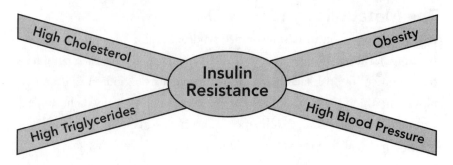

High Cholesterol — Obesity — Insulin Resistance — High Triglycerides — High Blood Pressure

Since Dr. Reaven's definition, the metabolic syndrome has been modified and expanded to include other risk factors. Instead of insulin resistance being classified as one of the *symptoms* of metabolic syndrome, current research views high insulin levels as the root *cause* for the syndrome and its coexisting conditions. These high insulin levels result from a high intake of refined carbohydrates coupled with insulin resistance. Therefore the X does not encompass the vast risk factors that now exist for metabolic syndrome.

The definition of metabolic syndrome now expands beyond the five conditions first defined and includes not only obesity, abnormal cholesterol, high blood pressure, and glucose intolerance, but also socioeconomic status, birth weight, genes, and inflammation as reasonable risks for the development of metabolic syndrome. Most people with metabolic syndrome have no idea they have it, and many experts say that unless steps are taken to aggressively identify and treat it, it is likely to spawn future epidemics of heart attacks, strokes, sleep apnea, liver disease, polycystic ovary syndrome (related to female infertility), depression, and mood disorders.

IDENTIFYING METABOLIC SYNDROME

But how do you recognize and identify metabolic syndrome? Dr. Reaven made his discovery by directly measuring the insulin sensitivity of his subjects, which is a very labor-intensive, expensive process. This is not a test that is routinely done by physicians, so the diagnosis of insulin resistance needs to be based on measuring the other parameters, or the so-called "petals" of the daisy.

The Metabolic Syndrome Daisy

In a recent paper on insulin resistance syndrome (also known as metabolic syndrome), the syndrome was compared with a daisy, where "each petal represents one of the risk factors manifested in metabolic syndrome, all united by a stem, which represents cardiovascular disease, and a leaf which is type 2 diabetes. Insulin resistance is the root." The growing conditions of the daisy are diet, physical activity, socioeconomic status, ethnicity, and age.

Normally we think of flowers, especially the daisy with its bright, positive image, as happy; in fact the daisy is one of my favorite flowers because it is so happy-looking. There is nothing like a vase of beautiful daisies to light up a room. However, in the case of metabolic syndrome, the root, insulin resistance, is unhealthy. We need to start with a healthy root or core to develop a healthy body; or in this case a healthy daisy. So although the daisy is living, it isn't thriving because of the negative growing conditions, causing the petals to wilt, and the stem to weaken. Now that you have seen the analogy of the daisy, you can think of your own body. We all have a core that makes us thrive. Unfortunately, because of what we eat and how we live, our core is suffering. In North America, we tend to eat dead food, the standard American diet (SAD) to feed a living body. You can live like this for a while, but sooner or later it will catch up with you. When it does, you will feel decreased energy, fall asleep at your desk mid-afternoon, have food cravings, fuzzy thinking, increasing weight around your middle, joint pain and aches, and later on disease conditions like heart disease and diabetes. Metabolic syndrome is just one of the results of a poor diet and lifestyle. We need to control the growing conditions of our body, so we can live and thrive, disease free. If we don't we will be like the metabolic syndrome daisy, with a weak stem and wilting petals.

Figure 1.4: The Metabolic Syndrome Daisy

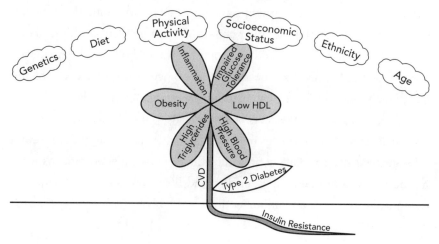

Figure 1.4 outlines the relationship between the growing conditions of the daisy, which include genetics, diet, physical inactivity, socioeconomic status, and birth weight, ethnicity, and age; the petals, which represent the risk factors (low HDL cholesterol, high triglycerides, inflammation, glucose intolerance, high blood pressure, and obesity), united by a stem and leaf, which is cardiovascular disease (CVD) and type 2 diabetes with insulin resistance as the root. This book is divided into sections related to each part of the daisy to help you fully understand how far-reaching and encompassing metabolic syndrome has become.

The key strategy in the prevention of insulin resistance and therefore metabolic syndrome (that is, to prevent future heart disease and diabetes) is to identify the presence of risk factors. The term "risk factor" refers to anything that might increase your chance of developing the disease. The higher the number of risk factors, the greater the likelihood that metabolic syndrome will develop. It is essential to identify the risk factors and then use the remaining chapters of this book, which includes dietary guidelines, lifestyle adjustments, and nutritional supplements to help reduce the risk factors and thereby prevent diabetes and heart disease.

INSULIN RESISTANCE

Insulin resistance is the root cause of metabolic syndrome. The Risk Assessment Quiz will help assess your risk factors for insulin resistance. It is possible to have insulin resistance without having metabolic syndrome (because you may not have developed the other conditions that go along with metabolic syndrome yet—see Table 1.2), but people with metabolic syndrome always have insulin resistance because insulin resistance is the root cause of the metabolic syndrome. If you catch insulin resistance in time, before it goes to far, you can reverse the effects before it leads to metabolic syndrome, and eventually type 2 diabetes. But once you have identified that you are insulin resistant, you need to take action immediately. Taking action means making necessary adjustments in your diet and lifestyle; these adjustments are expanded upon in the remaining sections of the book.

Insulin resistance can develop for a number of reasons, but primarily a diet rich in sugar, refined carbohydrates, and processed/convenience foods, combined with a sedentary lifestyle, are strong risk factors. The human body was not designed to handle the amount of refined sugar, fat, and other harmful foods that we are consuming. This type of diet can result in insulin resistance—that is, the body's tissues not responding normally to insulin. As a result, insulin levels become elevated by the body's attempt to overcome the resistance to insulin. High insulin levels leads to impaired glucose tolerance, obesity, high blood pressure, high triglycerides, high cholesterol, and inflammation (Insulin resistance will be discussed in more detail in Chapter 7.)

ASSESS YOUR RISK FOR METABOLIC SYNDROME

The following quiz will help you determine whether you have metabolic syndrome. You may have to visit your physician to find out your cholesterol levels to accurately assess your metabolic syndrome risk. This quiz addresses the growing conditions and risk factors, or "petals" of the daisy, and will help you identify, then either prevent or treat metabolic syndrome before the symptoms go too far. If you meet the criteria for metabolic syndrome, you need to run, not walk, to do something about it. Metabolic syndrome may give a person five times the risk of diabetes and more than double the risk of heart disease.

If you have a family history of diabetes; if you take medication to control your blood pressure, cholesterol, or triglycerides; if you are overweight and have difficulty losing weight—combined with the insulin resistance risk factors—then you most certainly have metabolic syndrome. Metabolic syndrome is the label that modern science has chosen for a condition caused by poor dietary and lifestyle choices. However, weight loss significantly improves all aspects of metabolic syndrome. Increasing physical activity and making dietary changes by restricting sugar, refined carbohydrates, and certain fats will improve metabolic syndrome.

Risk Assessment Quiz

1. Do you have a family member (parent or sibling) with type 2 diabetes?

☐ Yes = 10 Points   ☐ No = 0 Points

2. Is your body mass index (BMI) greater than 30? (Please see page 88 for information on how to calculate your BMI.)

☐ Yes = 10 Points   ☐ No = 0 Points

3. Do you have a pot belly or carry more of your fat around your abdominal region than on your hips and thighs?

☐ Yes = 10 Points   ☐ No = 0 Points

4. Is your total cholesterol more than 200 mg/dl?

☐ Yes = 10 Points   ☐ No = 0 Points

5. Is your HDL cholesterol less than 40 mg/dl (men) and less than 50 mg/dl (women)?

☐ Yes = 10 Points   ☐ No = 0 Points

6. Do you have high blood pressure (systolic >135 mmHg/diastolic >85 mmHg)?

☐ Yes = 10 Points   ☐ No = 0 Points

7. Do you take drugs to control your cholesterol, triglycerides, or blood pressure?

☐ Yes = 10 Points   ☐ No = 0 Points

8. Have you been diagnosed with an inflammatory condition such as rheumatoid arthritis, eczema, psoriasis, asthma, inflammatory bowel disease, or fibromyalgia?

☐ Yes = 10 Points   ☐ No = 0 Points

9. Do you eat fast food or convenience food more than twice per week?

☐ Yes = 10 Points   ☐ No = 0 Points

10. Do you eat refined-sugar sweets like ice cream, candies, and cookies more than three times per week?

☐ Yes = 10 Points   ☐ No = 0 Points

11. Do you drink any regular soft drinks?

☐ Yes = 10 Points   ☐ No = 0 Points

12. Do you have cravings for carbohydrates such as bread and pasta or other sugar foods?

☐ Yes = 10 Points   ☐ No = 0 Points

13. Do you exercise or do regular activity at least 30 minutes, five times per week?

☐ Yes = – 10 Points   ☐ No = +10 Points

If you scored more than 90 points you almost certainly have metabolic syndrome.

If you scored between 65 and 90 you likely have metabolic syndrome.

If you scored between 50 and 65 you are at risk of metabolic syndrome.

If you scored between 35 and 50 it is unlikely you have metabolic syndrome, but you may have some degree of insulin resistance.

If you scored below 30, congratulations, you are on your way to health!

WHAT YOU HAVE LEARNED IN THIS CHAPTER

- Metabolic syndrome is a collection of symptoms that make someone prone to type 2 diabetes and cardiovascular disease. The term refers to a cluster of symptoms that includes glucose intolerance (poor blood sugar control), obesity, blood-fat abnormalities (high levels of cholesterol and triglycerides), high blood pressure, and inflammation, with high insulin levels (insulin resistance) being the cause. These risk factors lead to a five times greater chance of developing type 2 diabetes and doubling your chance of cardiovascular disease.

- Metabolic syndrome can be compared with a daisy, where "each petal represents one of the risk factors manifested in metabolic syndrome, all united by a stem, which represents cardiovascular disease, and a leaf which is type 2 diabetes. Insulin resistance is the root." The growing conditions of the daisy are genetics, diet, physical activity, socioeconomic status, ethnicity, and age.

- Insulin resistance can develop for a number of reasons, but primarily high insulin levels, a diet rich in sugar, refined carbohydrates, processed/convenience food, and a sedentary lifestyle are strong risk factors. We need to prevent and control insulin resistance to avoid metabolic syndrome.

In the next chapter we will learn how significant dietary changes from what our ancestors ate have led to the overfed, undernourished society we live in today. Getting back to the basics, like the Paleolithic diet of whole foods, fruits and vegetables, nuts and seeds, and lean protein, will help control insulin resistance and prevent metabolic syndrome.

PART II

GROWING CONDITIONS

Chapter 2

YOU ARE WHAT YOU EAT

Modern-day lifestyles are busy, full of stress, and seem to produce time conflicts more than ever. With time being so precious, it is no wonder that quick and easy foods are preferred over foods we need to prepare. As we face epidemic numbers of people with obesity, diabetes, and cardiovascular disease, many people have started to question the role our modern diet plays in our health. There is no doubt that when you compare what we eat today to what our parents or grandparents ate, the changes are enormous. It is very likely that our grandparents wouldn't recognize many of the foods we take for granted, and one wonders what would happen to Grandpa's cholesterol levels, body weight, and overall health if he were to eat the highly processed fast food that is a major part of our diets.

During the past fifty years, dietary changes have accelerated, pushing us even further from our evolutionary baseline diet. Refined carbohydrates—pastas, breads, cereals, and breakfast bars—now dominate the diet. Many foods also contain large amounts of varying forms of sugar, along with partially hydrogenated oils (vegetable oils processed to have some of the characteristics of saturated fats). This type of diet wreaks havoc on glucose and insulin levels. As a consequence, these cells become resistant (or insensitive) to insulin, and blood levels of glucose and insulin increase, setting the stage for metabolic syndrome, diabetes, heart disease, and other disorders.

The foods we consume daily affect our health more than anything else. The easiest way to take control of our health is to take control of what we eat.

The foods of today are nothing like the foods of the past. Modern foods are laced with nitrates, preservatives, soy additives, plant byproducts, etc., and are heavily processed. Our insufficient dietary fiber intake is a major concern. It has been only recently that the amount of fiber in our diets has decreased so rapidly. Most livestock are pampered with high-caloric feed, injected with hormones and antibiotics, and not allowed to graze, resulting in meat with different nutrients than those of wild game. Many of the modern foods touted as "healthy" didn't even exist in our ancestors' diet. It is important to realize that what the majority of people eat today is not optimized for our bodies, but optimized for convenience, taste, and preservation.

WHEN TECHNOLOGY EXCEEDS HUMANITY

Our knowledge and technologies have advanced at a tremendous pace, but our bodies are still in the Stone Age. We still have the genetic makeup of our Paleolithic ancestors. Our bodies have not been given the necessary time to efficiently utilize these new foods. It takes thousands upon thousands of years to adapt to the dietary changes we have incorporated in our modern diet in a relatively short period of time. This sudden change in diet can account for many of the diseases that plague modern society.

The Stone Age Diet

Four million years ago our ancestors' diets consisted mainly of wild meat, fish, plants, nuts, seeds, and berries.

What we refer to as the Paleolithic diet or Stone Age diet is comparable to the diet of pre-agricultural humans (1.5 million to 10,000 years B.C.) and includes lean meat, fish, vegetables, fruits, roots, and nuts, while avoiding cereals, dairy products, salt, processed fat, and sugar. The underlying rationale for this type of diet is that foods that were once available are healthier than those recently introduced (dairy products, cereals, trans fats, sugar, etc.), since the human digestive and metabolic systems were not designed for the latter group of foods. In many ways Paleolithic diets were more nutritious than our modern convenience-oriented diet.

Table 2.1: Paleolithic Diet Compared to Modern Diet

Minerals	2 x More
Fiber	4 –10 x More
Antioxidants	10 x More
Omega-3 Fat	50 x More
Lactic acid bacteria	10 x More
Protein	2 x More
Saturated Fat	10 x Less
Trans Fat	100 x Less
Sodium	10 x Less

Numerous scientific papers have evaluated the Paleolithic diet for its ability to prevent obesity and Western diseases. This diet is often high in protein, but not necessarily low in carbohydrate. A literature review in 2002 examined more than two hundred scientific journals in medicine, nutrition, biology, and anthropology and found increasing evidence suggesting that a Paleolithic diet based on lean meat, fish, vegetables, and fruit may be effective in the prevention and treatment of common Western diseases. Avoiding dairy products, margarine, oils, refined sugar, and cereals, which provide seventy percent or more of the dietary intake in North America, may be advisable. Atherosclerosis (hardening of the arteries), stroke, type 2 diabetes, and insulin resistance seem largely preventable by adopting a Paleolithic diet.

Today's Diet, Yesterday's Genes

Grain products and concentrated sugars were absent from human nutrition until the development of agriculture ten thousand years ago. In terms of genetics and our bodies' ability to adapt to dietary change, ten thousand years is a very short time. The agrarian society encouraged humans to settle down, to produce gardens and crops, and to domesticate animals.

The meat of more sedentary domesticated animals has more fat than that of wild animals. The growth of agrarian society marks the initial increase in our fat consumption.

The archeological record shows that a sharp decline in stature and health came with the change to the agricultural diet and lifestyle. Early hunter-gatherers in the Paleolithic period were four to six inches taller than early farmers in the agricultural era. The hunters had stronger bones, fewer cavities, and, barring accident, they lived longer. Hunter-gatherers were rarely obese and had low rates of autoimmune diseases like arthritis and diabetes.

In spite of overall poorer health, the farmers took over the world. How did this happen? Hunting and gathering work only for small groups of people. Chiefdoms, kingdoms, and states arose only after the advent of farming. A few people could produce food for many. Those freed up from the day-to-day search for food could become artisans, soldiers, and bureaucrats. A thousand soldiers supported by ten thousand slaves toiling in the fields became the new super weapon. These guys could whip any band of hunter-gatherers! The old-time hunter-gatherers were simply out-organized and not bred as well. As more and more land was used for crops, the animals and those who followed them were driven off and marginalized. By the nineteenth and twentieth centuries we could find hunter-gatherers only in the deserts, jungles, and remote places like the Arctic.

In spite of civilization and ten thousand years of farming, all of us still have the old hunter-gatherer DNA. There has not been enough time to adapt to our new diet. Studies of mitochondrial DNA show virtually no difference between the most diverse populations on the planet—groups that separated long before the advent of agriculture.

From Cave Dwellers to Condo Owners

The Industrial Revolution sparked another huge change in nutrition as more people left the farms to work in factories, thus increasing the need for store-bought food for those without access to food or time to produce their own. In 1800, the great majority (97%) of the world's population lived in rural areas.

By the year 2000, almost 76% lived in urban areas. Reliance on grocers to provide food, and the grocers' desire (for financial reasons) to reduce wasted food, paved the way for the highly processed and preserved foodstuffs we find on North American supermarket shelves today.

The changes over the past hundred years in the human environment have happened too quickly for evolution to keep up. We are nearly genetically identical to our hunter-gatherer ancestors, yet we live in overcrowded and polluted cities, have frequent contact with harsh chemicals, and consume processed foods that are relatively deficient in essential nutrients. Urban society is built on cheap food. Without cheap food, we cannot live in cities. City life is built on stable food that can be easily and quickly prepared. Rich societies eat diets that are furthest from the most natural for humans. In comparison to our ancestors, we eat hundreds of times more trans fats (harmful artificial fat that is linked to many diseases including cancer and heart disease), ten times more saturated fats, and on average each one of us consumes 150 pounds of sugar per year.

The ecological consequences of large-scale agriculture are severe. Forests are cut down to make room for crops. Topsoil is washed or blown away. Today, fertilizers and insecticides are dumped on the land by the ton to improve yield. Runoff from the fields turns our rivers and bays toxic, therefore polluting our water supply. The wild animals that once lived on the land are disappearing because they have nowhere safe to go.

Furthermore we have bred our plants to produce the biggest and sweetest (highest sugar content) fruits. A great example of this is the blueberry. Compare a wild blueberry to the modern grocery store blueberry and you will see a remarkable difference. The wild blueberry is small and contains little sugar. It takes a handful of wild berries to equal the sugar content of two or three large commercial blueberries. In that handful of wild berries you are also getting a far larger amount of antioxidants and nutrients than you would by eating commercial berries. Farmers don't cultivate and breed our plants to grow the most nutritious fruit, just the best-tasting fruit. The same is true for most of our modern foods.

Modern-Day Diet

Our food options have changed throughout the centuries. About 72% of the calories consumed by people in the United States and Canada are from foods that never existed in the Paleolithic diet: refined sugars, artificial sweeteners, white flour, high-fructose corn syrup, and shortening (trans fats). Are humans designed to thrive on Krispy-Kreme doughnuts, Cocoa Crisps, Twinkies, Pringles, Big Macs? Some scientists have suggested that the key to good health is to adopt some aspects of the preagricultural diet of our ancestors. By changing the type and balance of fat and carbohydrates in our diet, we may actually prevent some of today's modern diseases.

Our bodies are not designed to eat many of the agricultural foods in our present diet, such as bread, corn, beans, and potatoes. As a result, many of us eventually become obese or are more likely to suffer from inflammatory diseases like diabetes, heart disease, arthritis, and allergies. Degenerative disease is a silent epidemic. Coronary heart disease is the leading cause of death in the United States and Canada. About 58 million people in the United States have high blood pressure, a major risk factor for coronary heart disease. Approximately 16 million people in the United States and 1.5 million in Canada have type 2 diabetes, the severest form of which causes kidney damage, limb damage, and other cardiovascular damage. More than 60% of the population have a weight problem (BMI>25), and 34% of us are obese (BMI>30; see page 88 in Chapter 6 to determine your BMI).

Increasing numbers of children are obese. More than a quarter of the population has metabolic syndrome. Studies on the particular diets of populations around the world and the incidence of degenerative disease in those populations point to a strong link between diet and degenerative diseases.

Why should we be surprised that the kinds of foods we evolved with can protect us from degenerative disease? Why should we be surprised if a diet that meets or exceeds our caloric and protein needs, but does not have the kinds, proportions, and levels of fats, oils, minerals, vitamins, and phytochemicals that are abundant in a whole-plant and animal-food diet is implicated in degenerative disease? Isn't the slow onset of degenerative disease more likely as we move further from our ancestors' diet? Common sense tells us degenerative disease is less likely the more we eat the kinds and quantities of foods that our bodies were intended to eat, instead of the toxic foods we consume today.

FAT

Civilization has certainly changed our lifestyles, yet our basic bodily needs have not changed since the beginning of the human race. Due to lifestyle and dietary habits with fast food and convenience foods, the general public consumes a diet high in fats.

Years ago, there was only limited access to saturated fats from wild animals (whose fat also contained the essential fats omega-3 and omega-6, known as the "good fats"). They ate more nuts and seeds and vegetables, which contain enough of these essential fats for their bodies to manufacture saturated fats. Essential fat used to come from the intact leaves, roots, nuts, and seeds people gathered. The rather unstable polyunsaturated fats didn't go rancid because they were eaten in a whole-food state. Naturally present antioxidants protected the fat from oxidation. Some wild seeds have quite astonishing levels of antioxidants. These natural antioxidants are largely absent in highly processed food.

Good Fats: Good Ratio

Virtually all fats found in natural foods are basically mixtures of saturated, monounsaturated, and polyunsaturated fats in different proportions. What is the proper proportion of fat in a diet? To answer this correctly we must take a lesson from our prehistoric ancestors.

Fats comprise about 35 to 40 percent of Paleolithic calories and consisted mainly of monounsaturated and the polyunsaturated omega-3 and 6 fats. Saturated fats made up less than 40 percent of the fat supply. Currently the North American diet contains similar amounts of fats (35 to 40%), but the amounts of the various types of fats are very different. The main fats eaten today are saturated fat from fatty red meats and dairy products and trans fats from margarine and processed baked goods. Omega-3s from fatty fish, green leafy vegetables, and nuts and seeds are almost non-existent. The overabundance of saturated fat, the introduction of an entirely new type of fat (trans fat), and a major deficiency in omega-3 fats have resulted in some of the major health problems we are experiencing.

As well, the fat profile in grain-fed animals is different from grass-fed animals. The fat of grain-fed animals has less omega-3s and more omega-6s than grass-fed. This is because of the corn that is fed to the animals. This shift from feeding grass to feeding grain has partly led to the imbalance of fat in our food supply today. Instead of consuming the optimal 4:1 to 1:1 omega-6 to omega-3 ratio, we are now consuming a 20:1 ratio. This excess consumption of omega-6 has dire consequences, for example many of the degenerative diseases we are experiencing today. If we rely on grain-fed animals, margarines, and vegetable oils as a significant part of our diet, we are likely in a state of essential fatty acid deficiency/imbalance.

When Good Fat Turns Trans

The use of omega-6 vegetable oils is so far-reaching that practically every fried food and snack food available has been cooked in soybean, corn, sunflower, or canola oil. These oils are usually processed by hydrogenation, which creates trans fats. This changes the molecular structure so the fat will be good for frying foods at a high temperatures and will provide a lengthy shelf life in the grocery store. Trans fats give a pleasing texture to baked goods. But our bodies cannot recognize trans fats and they do not have the ability to break them down. For example, it takes more than a hundred days for the trans fats in a small order of French fries to be eliminated from the body. Unfortunately, these trans fats promote inflammation and can lead to obesity, diabetes, and cardiovascular disease.

REFINED SUGAR AND CARBOHYDRATES

Honey Combs, Pepsi, Twinkies, cookies, ice cream, white pasta, white rice, white bread—these are just a few examples of refined sugars that fill our cupboards today. Every North American consumes around 150 pounds of sugar per year. Starch and refined sugar have become the backbone of our diet, but starch and refined sugar provide empty calories. In contrast, early humans consumed no refined sugar—only sugar that came from natural foods like berries picked from the trees.

Over the course of a year, a hunter-gatherer would consume more than a hundred different species of fruits and vegetables. These foods provided more than one hundred grams of fiber daily. Today, fewer than nine percent of North Americans eat the recommended five daily servings of fruits and vegetables. Our fruits and vegetables have been hybridized to increase sugar and starch content, at the expense of fiber. Early humans thrived on high-fiber fruits, primitive forms of leafy vegetables, and root vegetables (such as yams and sweet potatoes), which contained abundant nutrition. They consumed four to ten times more fiber than we do. Since these foods are digested slowly and have a low glycemic index (see "Carbohydrates and the Glycemic Index" in Chapter 4), early humans avoided the problems of large amounts of glucose being dumped into the bloodstream at once. As we discussed in Chapter 1, exposure to large amounts of glucose loads (50 to 60% of calories in the modern diet) creates insulin resistance, leading to metabolic syndrome, and then later on to type 2 diabetes and cardiovascular disease.

Grains were not consumed by our ancestors. Modern-day humans have difficulty digesting grains properly. Notice that corn, wheat, and milk are our most common food allergens.

Forty percent of our adult population shows some allergic response to dairy. Wheat and corn allergies are common. Legumes give most of us at least minimal digestive disturbance, and some legumes are rendered digestible only through processing. Many of us, while not diagnosed as allergic to these foods, have stressed immune systems. A stressed immune system is the instigator of autoimmune disease.

Our systems are stressed by these "indigestible" foods because we have not yet adapted to the onslaught of starch that agriculturalism has imposed upon us.

PROTEIN

In a Paleolithic diet, protein makes up about 25 to 30 percent of calories and is derived almost exclusively from game animals (high in iron, B vitamins, and minerals, but low in fat) and fish. Fish is the best source of the long-chain omega-3s, eicosapentaenoic acid (EPA) and docosahexaenoic acid (DHA). The North American diet consists of only 10 to 15 percent protein, and that protein is derived from high-fat meats, grains, dairy products, and legumes. Thus both the amount and sources vary greatly between the two dietary practices. High-quality protein is essential to regulating blood sugar levels and to controlling insulin resistance. Protein is involved in the production of glucagon. Glucagon is a hormone that allows the body to burn stored fat and stored carbohydrates (glycogen) for energy. It helps counter high insulin levels. We must consume adequate amounts of protein if we want to prevent or reverse insulin resistance. Protein also plays a major role in the prevention of autoimmune disease (in which the body's immune system begins to turn on itself, causing prolonged inflammation and tissue damage) by helping strengthen the immune system. However, when foreign substances are introduced, such as new sources of proteins (dairy, grains, legumes), which our ancestors did not consume, they present the immune system with completely new protein fragments that are very problematic.

OTHER NUTRIENTS

During the Paleolithic era, micronutrient (vitamins, minerals, antioxidants) consumption was about three times that of today, since the diet was rich in fruits and vegetables. Vitamin consumption was about three times greater, because early humans ate lots of fruits and vegetables. The average salt intake was about ten times less than the average North American's consumption today. This overabundance of sodium along with very low consumption of most minerals and vitamins has, not surprisingly, serious consequences for health.

WHAT YOU HAVE LEARNED IN THIS CHAPTER

- The food we eat today is nothing like the food our ancestors ate.
- We consume a diet high in processed, refined carbohydrates and trans and saturated fats instead of a diet rich in whole fruits and vegetables, lean meat and fish, and oil-bearing seeds and nuts.
- This dietary shift has had significant consequences on the health of North Americans. Modern-day diseases have a direct link to the type of food we consume.
- We need to get back to the basic components of the Paleolithic diet.

In the next chapter we will take a more in-depth look at dietary fat and its consequences on insulin resistance, inflammation, obesity, and the metabolic syndrome.

Chapter 3

THE SKINNY ON FAT

One of the growing conditions for the metabolic syndrome daisy is dietary fat. The incidence of metabolic syndrome, obesity, type 2 diabetes, and cardiovascular disease has increased. At the same time, major changes in the type and amount of fats we consume have occurred over the past forty to fifty years, reflected in increases in saturated fat (from both animal sources and hydrogenated oils), trans fats, vegetables oils rich in omega-6s, and an overall decrease in the omega-3s.

Finding the balance of the dietary fats is the key. Why is this? Diets high in the wrong types of fat make insulin resistance worse by interfering with the burning of glucose and increasing insulin resistance. So what kinds of fats should we be consuming?

There are some fats that are necessary for the body to function and you should be including them in your diet. These are unsaturated fats, namely the essential fatty acids. Then there are the bad fats that most of us eat every day, which increase our risk of heart disease, diabetes, metabolic syndrome, and inflammation. It is important to understand which fats you should avoid and which fats should be included in your meals in order to prevent insulin resistance and metabolic syndrome.

There are two main groups of fats—saturated and unsaturated.

SATURATED FATS: THE GOOD, THE NOT-SO-BAD, THE BAD, AND THE UGLY

Saturated fats are semisolid at room temperature and are found in animal products, such as red meat, pork, and lamb, and dairy products like milk, cheese, and butter, as well as in processed foods. They are generally considered "bad" fats, as they can contribute to heart disease; therefore most health authorities recommend reducing saturated fats in the diet.

However, not all saturated fats are created equally. There are three subgroups of saturated fats based on their chain length: short-chain, medium-chain, and long-chain fats.

The Good

Short-chain saturates, found in butter, coconut oil, and palm kernel oil, do not clog arteries, nor do they cause heart disease. Rather, they are easily digested and a source of fuel for energy.

The Not-So-Bad

Medium-chain saturates are found in several different foods, but the highest content (just as in short-chain saturates) is found in palm kernel and coconut oil. Medium-chain saturates are not associated with increasing cholesterol levels or the occurrence of heart disease. Medium-chain triglycerides (MCT oils) are used by athletes and dieters who want to convert fat into energy rather than store it as fat.

The Bad

Long-chain saturates are the "bad" fats associated with raising LDL (the bad cholesterol), lowering HDL (the good cholesterol), and increasing the risk of metabolic syndrome by causing insulin resistance and heart disease. The bad saturated fats are found in meat. Long-chain saturates are also a by-product of hydrogenation, a process that turns a liquid fat (at room temperature) into a solid and is employed in the manufacture of most margarines and shortening. Long-chain saturates are also abundant in restaurant fried foods, junk food, packaged baked goods, and processed foods. Hydrogenation or partial hydrogenation also distorts the fatty acids into a more poisonous form—trans fats.

The Ugly

Trans fat is by far the worst type of fat. Numerous research studies have shown that trans fats are more damaging to the heart than are saturated fats. The Institute of Medicine declared there is no safe level of trans fats and that consumption should be reduced as much as possible.

Trans fats were developed when there was a backlash against saturated fats. They are artificial, formed by a process of high temperature and hydrogenation that turns refined oils into margarines, shortenings, and partially hydrogenated vegetable oils, making them solid or semisolid and "shelf stable." Our bodies cannot recognize them as nutrients and therefore are not able to process them. They are, however, a food manufacturer's dream as they are inexpensive to produce and extend the shelf life of foods.

Trans fats are found everywhere in your cupboard, yet I would bet most of you don't even know you are eating them. Trans fats have been dubbed "phantom fats" because, until recently, the labeling of trans fats was not mandatory. Thankfully, now you can pick up a box of crackers and see what the trans fat content is, then make the right decision for your heart and waistline and put the crackers back on the shelf if they contain trans fats.

The typical North American consumes between eight and thirteen grams of trans fats per day. Trans fats are found in forty percent of the food on our grocery store shelves. For example, if you have the typical breakfast of a coffee and doughnut, you consume 3.2 grams of trans fats when you eat the doughnut. If you are like most people who don't have enough time to pack a lunch, and if you are busy running errands at noon, you stop and eat fast food. You will be getting 6.8 grams of trans fats from your large order of French fries. You are at 10 grams of trans fats, and you haven't even made it past lunch

Table 3.1: Trans Fat Content of Some Common Foods (in grams)

Vegetable Shortening	1.4 – 4.2
Margarine (stick)	1.8 – 3.5
Margarine (tub, regular)	0.4 – 1.6
Salad Dressings (regular)	0.06 – 1.1
Vegetable Oils	0.01 – 0.06
Pound cake	4.3
Doughnuts	0.3 – 3.8
Microwave Popcorn	2.2
Chocolate Chip Cookies	1.2 – 2.7
French Fries (fast food)	0.7 – 3.6
Snack Crackers	1.8 – 2.5

SATURATED, TRANS FATS AND METABOLIC SYNDROME

Did you know that each gram of trans fats increases your risk of heart disease by twenty percent? And then we wonder why cardiovascular disease is the number one killer in both Canada and the United States, when trans fat consumption is between eight and thirteen grams per day.

Trans fats promote obesity and insulin resistance because our bodies can't recognize them, as they are shaped differently from natural fats, such as unsaturated fats. Trans fats crowd out the essential fats from the cells. Polyunsaturated fats determine the fluidity of the cell. When there are fewer essential fats, the cell becomes rigid and hard, thereby reducing the number and sensitivity of insulin receptors. When insulin receptors become less sensitive to insulin, blood glucose levels remain high, leading to type 2 diabetes. In one study, women who ate margarine (which contains trans fats) four or more times per week had a higher than normal risk of three of the symptoms of metabolic syndrome: high triglycerides, low HDL cholesterol, and high total cholesterol. Trans fats increase the size of fat cells, and large fat cells have fewer insulin receptors and store more fat than normal fat cells. The health and dollar impact of trans fats is enormous, and the government is hoping that the new trans fat regulation will save $5 billion in health care costs in Canada over the next 20 years by helping people trim their waistlines and reduce diabetes, coronary heart disease, and stroke.

A study done in June 2005 at the University of Alberta discovered that people with a high-fat diet, or those who are overweight, may be at increased risk of developing type 2 diabetes. The study, published in *Diabetes*, suggested that saturated and trans fats are much more effective activators of a specific potassium channel found in the pancreas. When activated, this channel reduces insulin secretion from the pancreas and increases blood sugar levels, increasing the risk of type 2 diabetes. Polyunsaturated fats are poor activators of the potassium channel.

If you want to prevent insulin resistance and the very serious complications associated with it, you should substantially reduce your intake of trans fats. This can be done by reading labels to determine the trans fat content in that food product. Typical foods containing trans fats include packaged and convenience foods like chips, crackers, cookies, commercial baked goods, and fast food.

GOOD FATS: ESSENTIAL FATTY ACIDS

Unsaturated Fats

There are three major classes of unsaturated fats: omega-3, omega-6, and omega-9. The omega-3s and omega-6s are polyunsaturated and they are an essential part of the diet because the body cannot make them. The omega-9s (found in olive oil) are monounsaturated and nonessential (the body can make them from other fats.) Yet they are still a very healthy type of fat, and one that a person with or at risk of metabolic syndrome should emphasize in the diet.

Unsaturated fats are liquid at room temperature and are generally considered to be "good" fats. Typically, the more liquid a fat is, the healthier it is. Unsaturated fats can be further classified as monounsaturated or polyunsaturated. Monounsaturated fats remain liquid at room temperature, but solidify in colder temperatures. A great example of a monounsaturated fat is olive oil, rich in heart-healthy omega-9s known as oleic acid. What happens to olive oil when you put it in the fridge? It turns cloudy. This is because of the monounsaturated fats in the olive oil. Olive oil has been found to help addressing insulin resistance and achieve healthier cholesterol levels.

Polyunsaturated fats are liquid at room temperature and remain liquid in colder temperatures. Sources of polyunsaturated fats include black currant, borage, evening primrose, corn, flaxseed, safflower, sunflower, sesame, soy, fish oil, fatty fish, nuts, and seeds. However, the only polyunsaturated fats I recommend are from fatty wild fish, fish oil, flax seeds and flax oil, borage and evening primrose oil, and all nuts and seeds. The other sources mentioned have an imbalance of the omega-6 fats and have undergone tremendous processing and refinement, making them unhealthy and toxic.

Understanding EFAs: Why Essential Fats Are So Essential

Essential fatty acids are polyunsaturated fats that include:

- The omega-6 fatty acid linoleic acid (LA) and its metabolites, gamma linolenic acid (GLA) and arachidonic acid (AA).
- The omega-3 fatty acid alpha linolenic acid (ALA) and its metabolites, eicosapentaenoic acid (EPA) and docosahexaenoic acid (DHA).

Theoretically, only LA and ALA are absolutely essential. However, the fatty acids derived from them are also generally considered essential. Deficiencies in EFAs are common today for three reasons: modern dietary and lifestyle choices; the effects of environmental pollution; and because some people have trouble converting LA and ALA to their metabolites (metabolites are responsible for hormone production). An EFA deficiency or imbalance is a serious problem that can eventually lead to insulin resistance and metabolic syndrome.

Functions of EFAs

The three main functions of EFAs are to regulate cellular processes, influence membrane function and integrity, and produce hormones that regulate and balance inflammation.

Regulating Cellular Processes and Cell Membrane Integrity

EFAs are integral components of cell membranes, determining fluidity and other physical properties as well as affecting structural functions, for example, the maintenance of enzyme activity. Our bodies are built of billions of cells. Cells are built of membranes, and membranes are built of fats. Cell membranes built with polyunsaturated, essential fats are less rigid and more fluid than membranes built with saturated fats. Fluid cells are extremely important as they allow the transport of valuable nutrients into the cells; they help keep toxins out of the cells; they elasticize tissue; they expand blood vessel walls to reduce heart workload; and they improve the overall function of organs.

Figure 3.1: Cell Membrane Fluidity

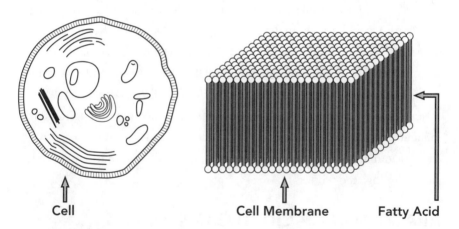

Cell   Cell Membrane   Fatty Acid

If your cells are built of saturated fats, they will become rigid and hard. You may not notice the effects of your diet and its role in health when you are young, but if you continue to consume a diet full of unhealthy fats, you will start to see the effects manifested in inflammatory conditions like arthritis, insulin resistance, metabolic syndrome, cardiovascular disease, and diabetes. It is extremely important that your cells are built of healthy fats, which keep the cells fluid. Fluid cells influence insulin sensitivity; they help your body utilize the insulin produced by your pancreas, and they help control your body's glucose levels.

The Power of Hormones

Some of the most potent effects of EFAs are related to their conversion into a series of eicosanoids, or hormones. They are intracellular communication agents that control the balance of virtually every system in the body, including the mechanisms for inflammation, blood clotting, and blood vessel dilation. They include, but are not limited to, anti-inflammatory and inflammatory prostaglandins (PGE series 1, 2, 3) and other immune system responders such as thromboxanes, leukotrienes, and hydroxy fatty acids.

LINOLEIC ACID: THE OMEGA-6 PARENT

EFAs control the breakdown and use of hormones through a metabolic pathway in our bodies. Under optimal conditions, the body processes linoleic acid, one of the two primary essential fatty acids needed for health, through a series of steps that eventually leads to the production of hormones. The diagram "The Metabolic Pathway for LA" shows how LA produces GLA with the help of the delta-6 desaturase, or D6D enzyme. Another enzyme, elongase, creates dihomo-gamma linolenic acid (DGLA). After one more reaction, the result is PGE1 and 15-hydroxy DGLA, the hormones that reduce inflammation, dilate blood vessels, and inhibit blood clotting. Their strong anti-inflammatory properties help the body recover from injury by reducing pain, swelling, and redness.

ARACHIDONIC ACID: THE OMEGA-6 INFLAMMATORY VILLAIN

Arachidonic acid (AA) is another omega-6 fat that produces hormones. The AA hormones work completely differently than the DGLA hormones, although they are both part of the omega-6 family. The hormones produced by AA include the five families of leukotrienes (LTA4, LTB4, LTD4, LTE4, LTF4) and the "2" family of prostaglandins (TXA2, PGD2, PGE2, PGF2a, PGI2). There are many types of inflammatory messengers, but prostaglandins and leukotrienes are the central players that can be controlled through diet. The major pro-inflammatory mediators are AA (which enhances platelet stickiness), TXA2 (which constricts the blood vessels, increases platelet stickiness, and induces cytokine production), and LTB4 (which promotes white blood cell attraction, adhesion, and activation). The properties of these mediators are important when the body suffers from a wound or injury; without them you could bleed to death if you cut yourself. However, a variety of dietary and lifestyle factors can lead to an excess production of the hormones from AA. North Americans tend to eat too much AA acid from red meat, eggs, farmed salmon, and shellfish, whereas those who follow a Stone Age or vegetarian diet will have more moderate and healthier levels of AA.

Excessive dietary intake of AA is a huge problem in North America that leads to excessive inflammation. What is the source of the numerous inflammatory conditions now prevalent? One of the main culprits is an imbalance of the fats, primarily excessive AA consumption, and a deficiency of the anti-inflammatory omega-3s and the anti-inflammatory omega-6 GLA. But can we stop the AA pathway from producing inflammatory prostaglandins? The answer is yes, with dietary changes.

AA, INSULIN RESISTANCE, AND INFLAMMATION

Many people with metabolic syndrome have a dietary status in which the eicosanoid (hormone) pathways are driven toward the production of pro-inflammatory hormones. This may occur as a consequence of dietary deficiency of certain polyunsaturated fats, or as a consequence of alterations in the ratio of omega-6 and omega-3. There is evidence that insulin sensitivity and excessive consumption of dietary arachidonic acid are linked to inflammation. Studies show that essential fatty acids can affect the release of insulin. The insulin-releasing effect of fats decreases with the degree of unsaturation, meaning the more saturated a fat is, the less chance the pancreas has of releasing insulin, which is why the polyunsaturated fats do a better job of enabling insulin secretion.

A diet rich in omega-3 polyunsaturated fats has been shown to reduce the risk for developing diabetes in healthy women. Diets that are higher in the omega-6, linoleic, and arachidonic acid, and in trans fats, and lower in omega-3 content, have been linked to increasing rates of insulin resistance and type 2 diabetes. Linoleic acid and arachidonic acid prevent the omega-3s from producing anti-inflammatory hormones. The increased proportion of omega-6 fatty acids in the Western diet has risen as fats from fish, wild game, and leaves were replaced by linoleic and arachidonic acid from seeds and oils. Changes in feeding livestock and poultry have also altered the omega-6–omega-3 content of meat.

Numerous theories have been suggested for the relationship between fats and insulin resistance, including changes in membrane fluidity (that is, the poly-unsaturated fats make the cells more fluid compared to saturated and trans fats, which create rigid, hard cells), the number of insulin receptor sites, and the increased activity of insulin receptors (that is, polyunsaturated fats make the insulin receptor sites more active). Research has shown that as the omega-6–omega-3 ratio decreases, insulin resistance improves. The anti-inflammatory properties of omega-3s also improve insulin sensitivity brought about by inflammation.

By decreasing the levels of inflammatory omega-6s and increasing the dietary content of anti-inflammatory omega-3s, we can improve insulin sensitivity and thus prevent metabolic syndrome. The use of omega-3s and the omega-6 GLA is really twofold: studies show they prevent and treat the unwanted outcomes of metabolic syndrome, namely diabetes and heart disease. Achieving the correct dietary ratio of these fatty acids will decrease inflammation, which will reverse and treat metabolic syndrome, and it will also decrease existing inflammation in those who suffer from other modern chronic diseases.

Figure 3.2: Omega-6 Fatty Acids Pathway

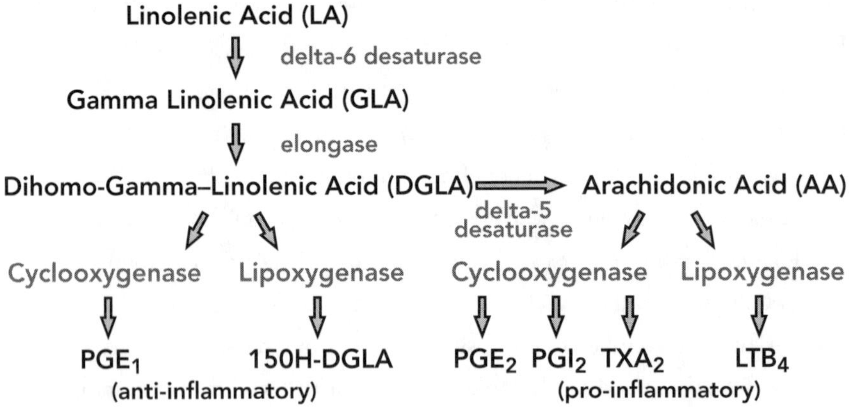

Linolenic Acid (LA)

⇩ delta-6 desaturase

Gamma Linolenic Acid (GLA)

⇩ elongase

Dihomo-Gamma–Linolenic Acid (DGLA) ⟹ **Arachidonic Acid (AA)**

delta-5 desaturase

Cyclooxygenase   Lipoxygenase   Cyclooxygenase   Lipoxygenase

⇩   ⇩   ⇩   ⇩   ⇩   ⇩

PGE_1 150H-DGLA PGE_2 PGI_2 TXA_2 LTB_4
(anti-inflammatory)   (pro-inflammatory)

Alpha-Linolenic Acid: The Omega-3 Parent

The body processes alpha-linolenic acid (ALA) in much the same way as it does linoleic acid, as you can see in Figure 3.3. However, the D6D enzyme has a higher attraction for ALA than for LA; it will convert ALA into its metabolites before it will break down LA. The primary goal of ALA is to be converted into eicosapentaenoic acid (EPA) and docosahexaenoic acid (DHA). Omega-3s from plants and fish reduce the levels of pro-inflammatory compounds from AA, thereby increasing insulin sensitization.

The important hormone derived from EPA is PGE3, which is beneficial against trauma and infection because, if required, it can be both anti-inflammatory and pro-inflammatory. However, because of the excessive inflammation we experience in North America, EPA has become known and used as a potent anti-inflammatory agent. This is the basis of the anti-inflammatory action of the omega-3 fatty acids—competing with pro-inflammatory AA hormones and reducing their levels—as well as the independent benefits of omega-3s for insulin sensitivity. EPA has been shown to enhance insulin sensitivity through effects on PPAR-receptors, which regulate the actions of insulin. The problem is the relative deficiency of this important fat in the diet.

Recent findings demonstrate that EPA is a precursor to resolvin, a potent bioactive mediator, which possesses both anti-inflammatory and protective properties. It is biosynthesized by new pathways triggered by aspirin and omega-3s. Resolvins inhibit both the migration of inflammatory cells to sites of inflammation and the turning on of other inflammatory cells.

Most of us do not have a healthy balance of these dietary fats; this good-fat deficiency can lead to many diseases. The typical North American diet contains too much saturated and trans fats and an overabundance of arachidonic acid, but is deficient in the anti-inflammatory omega-6 GLA and the omega-3s EPA and DHA.

Figure 3.3: Omega-3 Metabolic Pathway

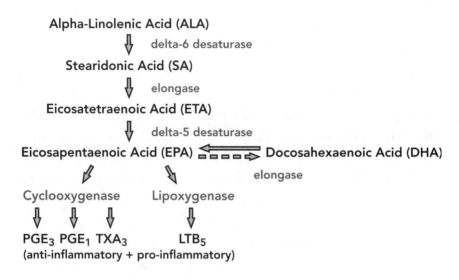

Enzyme Impairment

Both LA (omega-6) and ALA (omega-3) require the D6D enzyme to begin the first step in the reaction, a slow step known as the "rate-limiting step." Without the action of the D6D enzyme, the pathway is blocked and the production of good hormones is altered. There are numerous lifestyle and environmental factors that can impair the D6D enzyme, including:

- A high intake of saturated and trans fats
- A high intake of LA (from refined grocery-store vegetable oils such as corn, canola, sunflower, and safflower)
- Some pharmaceutical drugs and food additives
- Excess alcohol consumption
- Smoking
- Stress
- Advancing age (as we grow older, the enzyme becomes less effective)
- Infant prematurity (D6D enzyme does not become very efficient until about six months of age)

- Allergy-related eczema
- Diabetes
- Cancer
- Viral infections

A deficiency of the D6D enzyme results in a hormonal imbalance that can have serious health effects. Inflammation, blood vessel constriction, increased allergic response, impaired immune response, and abnormal cell function may result. In fact, an overwhelming number of diseases affecting us today are associated with this imbalance: arthritis, diabetic nerve damage, heart attacks, high blood pressure, atherosclerosis, insulin resistance, metabolic syndrome, allergies, and skin inflammation.

How can we overcome impaired enzymes to prevent hormonal imbalances? Impaired enzymes cannot be fixed, but they can be bypassed by supplementing the diet with the healthy EFAs that don't require the D6D enzyme for processing. For example, a diet high in fatty fish would supply the body with EPA without having to follow the reaction process to receive the beneficial hormones. It would be a direct source of the anti-inflammatory hormones that your body requires.

HOW TO BALANCE YOUR OMEGA-6s AND OMEGA-3s

Optimal fat ratios are important to increase the omega-3 and omega-6 content of body tissues. Increasing the good fat in the body will help decrease the "bad" saturated and trans fats linked to insulin resistance and metabolic syndrome. While all EFAs are crucial for our diet, it is important to ensure that we balance the omega-3s and omega-6s.

The typical North American diet provides an astonishing 20:1 to 30:1 ratio of omega-6 to omega-3. It's no wonder we are facing serious health problems today, especially as our ancestors consumed a diet with a 1:1 ratio. We are getting approximately twenty times the level of omega-6s we once did. Where is all this omega-6 coming from? Refined, grocery-store vegetable oils—corn, canola, safflower, and sunflower—and grain-fed meat are common contributors. There is no consensus yet on what the ideal amount or ratio of these EFAs should be in the human diet. However, it is clear that the ratio is much higher than it once was, suggesting we need to get back to consuming a ratio of 1:1 to 4:1 as our ancestors did. The unbalanced ratio of the modern Western diet promotes insulin resistance, leading to obesity, metabolic syndrome, and type 2 diabetes, because our cells cannot function with the excessive omega-6. In one study of overweight individuals the most insulin-sensitive people were those who had higher omega-3 levels and lower C-reactive protein (another sensitive indicator of inflammation) than those with insulin resistance. Our bodies were not designed to utilize refined omega-6s. We need to get back to the basics and eat more sources of omega-3s such as green leafy vegetables, nuts and seeds, wild fatty fish, and other healthy oils like avocado and olive oils.

OMEGA-3s IMPROVE METABOLIC SYNDROME RISK FACTORS

Research with the Greenland Eskimos showed that fish oil may protect against diabetes. Nutrition researchers at Pennington Biomedical Research Institute showed that three months of daily supplementation with DHA produced a clinically significant improvement in insulin sensitivity in overweight study participants.

In one study, twelve overweight men and women aged forty to seventy consumed 1.8 grams of DHA at breakfast for twelve weeks. None of the study participants had diabetes, but they all suffered from insulin resistance. Using blood tests taken at the start and end of the study, the researchers assessed changes in each person's insulin resistance.

They saw a change in insulin sensitivity after the twelve weeks of DHA supplementation. Seventy percent of the study participants showed an improvement in insulin-related function, and in fifty percent there was clinically significant change.

A recent U.S. government-sponsored review of the scientific literature showed positive news for people with metabolic syndrome: omega-3s from fish and fish oil reduced triglyceride levels (one of the risk factors for metabolic syndrome). The omega-3s also help keep arteries from narrowing in people with high cholesterol levels. Omega-3s are powerful anti-inflammatory agents. Inflammation is a risk factor for the development of metabolic syndrome.

Other research has found omega-3s to be powerful weight-loss agents, helping overweight individuals shed unwanted pounds. Overweight people are at a greater risk of developing metabolic syndrome. One twelve-week intervention trial studied the effects of omega-3s from fish oil in combination with aerobic exercise three times a week. Study participants were overweight and had metabolic syndrome. The results showed that the total proportion of fat in the body, particularly in the abdominal region, was reduced significantly in the fish-oil-plus-exercise group, but not by fish oil alone or exercise alone. The researchers concluded that omega-3s in fish oil can switch on enzymes specifically involved in oxidizing or burning fat, but they need a driver (exercise) to increase the metabolic rate to lower body fat. The researchers confirmed seven ways in which omega-3s help with weight loss:

- Fish oil omega-3s stimulate secretion of leptin, a hormone that decreases appetite and promotes the burning of fat.
- Fish oil omega-3s enable burning of dietary fats by helping the body move fatty acids into body cells for burning as fuel.
- Fish oil omega-3s encourage the body to store dietary carbohydrates in the form of glycogen, rather than as hard-to-lose body fat.
- Fish oil omega-3s reduce inflammation, which is known to promote weight gain.
- Fish oil omega-3s enhance blood sugar control by increasing the insulin-producing cells' sensitivity to sugar.
- Fish oil omega-3s flip off genetic switches that promote inflammation and storage of food as body fat.
- Fish oil omega-3s help the body transport glucose from blood to cells by increasing the fluidity of the cell membranes.

In summary, the researchers concluded that omega-3s are one of the best dietary weight-control aids discovered to date. The results of this new Australian study indicate that combining omega-3s with moderate aerobic exercise yields a synergistic effect that surpasses the weight control and body composition benefits of each.

GOOD FOODS WITH GOOD FATS

Healthy fats are easily consumed from a variety of delicious sources. Avocadoes, dark green leafy vegetables, fatty fish, nuts and seeds, olives, and unrefined expeller-pressed oils are rich in essential fatty acids and can protect you from obesity, insulin resistance, metabolic syndrome, and the consequences—diabetes and heart disease.

Ways to Increase Good Fats in Your Diet

- Eat cold-water, fatty fish such as wild salmon, tuna, mackerel, sardines, or anchovies two times per week. The American Heart Association recommends this to prevent heart disease. If you don't like the taste of fish, try a toxin-free fish oil supplement containing at least 500 mg of omega-3s. Aim for one gram of omega-3s per day. The American Heart Association recommends up to 3 grams of omega-3s per day to lower triglycerides, one of the risk factors, or "petals," of metabolic syndrome.
- Consume a GLA supplement, for example borage oil, to ensure levels of the anti-inflammatory omega-6.
- Flax seeds are the best sources of omega-3s in the plant kingdom.
- Eat nuts like walnuts, brazil nuts, butter nuts, macadamia nuts.
- The more green the better. The dark green leafy vegetables are good sources of omega-3s. Try romaine lettuce, mixed greens, spirulina, purslane, kale, Swiss chard, and arugula.
- Make your own salad dressing using flax oil. (See recipe for Dijon Flax Dressing, page 46.)
- Avoid refined grocery-store oils, for example canola, safflower, and sunflower. These oils are heavily processed and contain an abundance of omega-6,

which can lead to insulin resistance. Use extra virgin olive oil, coconut oil, and macadamia nut oil as your primary cooking oils.

- Make "Better Butter" by combining flax oil or other EFA rich oils with your butter. Use as a spread. (See recipe on page 46.)
- When possible, consume free-range meat, which contains higher levels of omega-3s than grain-fed meat. The grain fed to the animals is rich in omega-6s, which changes the fatty acid profile of the meat and leads to the imbalance of fats.

Table 3.1: Food Sources of Saturated and Unsaturated Fats

Saturated	Animal based foods including red meat, butter, milk, cheese. Leaner cuts of meat like chicken and turkey contain saturated fats but to a lesser degree. For further clarification on saturated fats see chapter 3.
Trans	Hydrogenated oils, margarines, and processed and convenience foods such as baked goods, chips, crackers, cookies, and cold cereals. Look for the words "hydrogenated" and "partially hydrogenated" on food labels.
Monounsaturated	Mediterranean diet is full of the omega-9 monounsaturated fats. This includes olive oil, avocadoes, macadamia nut oil, walnuts, almonds, flax seeds, and hemp seeds.
Polyunsaturated Omega-3	Free-range meat (contains the omega-3 alpha linolenic acid), green leafy vegetables such as romaine lettuce, mixed greens, spirulina, kale, spinach, Swiss chard, arugula, nuts, and seeds (almonds, walnuts, soybeans, hemp seeds, and flax seeds). The longer chain omega-3s are found in fatty, cold-water fish including salmon, mackerel, and tuna.
Polyunsaturated Omega-6	Vegetable oils such as canola, corn, safflower, and sunflower oil. Margarines are made from these oils, as well as many processed and convenience foods. Look for the words "linoleic acid" and "polyunsaturated omega-6," which indicate this type of fat. We have an overabundance of these fats in our diet, therefore we need to reduce our consumption.

Dijon Flax Dressing

3 tbsp red wine vinegar
2 tsp honey
4 shallots, finely minced
2 tbsp ground flax seeds
1/2 cup flax oil or a combination of flax and olive oils

Combine all the dressing ingredients and shake well. Taste and adjust with salt and pepper to suit your preference.

Better Butter Recipe

Cut 1 lb unsalted butter into eight pieces. Put butter and 1 cup high-quality EFA-rich oil into the food processor and blend until smooth. Spoon into a covered container and refrigerate. Not only will you have better butter, but it will remain soft even though refrigerated. Makes 2 cups.
Recipe originally appeared in *Healthy Immunity*

CONJUGATED LINOLEIC ACID (CLA): THE NEW KID ON THE BLOCK

Conjugated linoleic acid, which is necessary for cell growth and as a building block of cell membranes and has been shown to reduce body fat and increase lean body mass in both humans and animals, occurs naturally in dairy foods and grass-fed beef and lamb. It is produced by the intestinal bacteria of animals when they convert omega-6 linoleic acid into CLA. Humans cannot convert linoleic acid into CLA, so we must rely on the foods we eat, or on supplementation, to acquire necessary amounts of CLA. Unfortunately, the CLA content of dairy and meat products has declined in the past few decades because of increased antibiotic use in cattle and changes in the livestock's food from grass to grain. To illustrate, Australian cows have three to four times as much CLA in their meat as American cows. Most Americans have inadequate amounts of CLA in their diet. The introduction of low-fat and non-fat milk has also contributed to the relative deficiency of CLA in the Western diet. It is the fat content of milk that contains CLA. Could this deficiency of CLA be partly to blame for the epidemic of overweight people?

CLA for Lean Bodies

To date there are more than five hundred published research studies supporting CLA's ability to exert positive effects on fat loss, prevent and control type 2 diabetes, protect against heart disease, reduce the risk of atherosclerosis, and modulate the immune response.

Early research in 1951 paved the way for groundbreaking research on CLA and fat loss in humans. The first human clinical trial using CLA was conducted in 1997 in Norway and published in the *Journal of Nutrition* in 2000. The 90-day double-blind, randomized, placebo-controlled trial investigated the effects of CLA on different diseases. Control groups were compared to those receiving 1.7 g to 6.8 g per day. Results showed that 3.4 g of CLA per day is enough to obtain all the beneficial effects on body fat, while the group given the highest dose of 6.8 g of CLA per day also experienced the increase in lean body mass. In fact, the CLA group achieved a remarkable twenty percent decrease in body fat and an average loss of seven pounds of fat without changing their diet.

CLA Stops Fat from Coming Back

In August 2000, the results of a trial designed to assess the effects of CLA on body composition of obese men and women were released. Eighty overweight people took part in the six-month study in which they dieted and exercised. As expected, most people initially lost weight, but once their diets ended, many regained some of the weight. The participants who were not given CLA put pounds back in a fat-to-lean muscle mass ratio of 75:25, which is typical for most people. Those subjects who took CLA regularly regained less fat and retained more muscle mass with an impressive, statistically significant ratio of 50:50.

CLA and Exercise: Lose Fat More Quickly

Does CLA influence the effects of exercise? A Norwegian study published in 2001 in *The Journal of International Medical Research* says that it does. This trial focused on twenty people recruited from a physical fitness center where they participated in regular physical training consisting of ninety minutes of strenuous exercise three times a week.

The study showed that those participants who ingested 1.8 g of CLA per day for twelve weeks experienced significant body fat reduction when compared to the control group. The control group continued to exercise, but were given a placebo instead of CLA. CLA reduced body fat, but because lean muscle was increased, there was no actual change in body weight.

CLA Improves Insulin Sensitivity

CLA will help to reduce body fat, which will in turn improve insulin resistance. In animal studies, CLA has demonstrated an outstanding ability to prevent and control type 2 diabetes by sensitizing insulin. Researchers from Purdue University in Indiana reported a dramatic improvement in insulin response in patients taking 6 g of CLA per day. The eight-week trial involved twenty-two subjects. More than 64 percent of the patients experienced an improvement in their leptin levels. Leptin is a hormone that regulates both insulin and weight gain. These results suggest that CLA can help prevent or delay the onset of diabetes.

In conclusion, a deficiency of dietary CLA may be a major factor in causing Americans to gain so many fat pounds and develop insulin resistance. Luckily CLA is available today as a convenient dietary supplement. CLA is a potent insulin sensitizer; it lowers insulin resistance, and consequently insulin levels. By activating certain enzymes and enhancing glucose transport into the cells, CLA lowers blood sugar levels and normalizes insulin levels.

WHAT YOU HAVE LEARNED IN THIS CHAPTER

- There has been a significant shift in the type of fat consumed in our modern-day diet. Trans and saturated fats are abundant, leading to insulin resistance.
- There is an overabundance of omega-6 linoleic acid and arachidonic acid. These fatty acids produce pro-inflammatory prostaglandins, which can lead

to insulin resistance and decrease the production of anti-inflammatory prostaglandins from omega-3s. We need to increase our consumption of fish-based omega-3s to help decrease insulin resistance.

• CLA content in our diet has been depleted, but there are supplements that can provide the benefit of fat loss, increased muscle mass, and improved insulin sensitivity.

In the next chapter we will look at the effects of carbohydrates on developing insulin resistance and metabolic syndrome.

Chapter 4

CARBOHYDRATE CRAZY

J ust as the wrong types of fat in our diet contribute to insulin resistance, so do the wrong types of carbohydrates. We've come a long way since the days when one of the knee-jerk answers to the question "What should I eat to help me lose weight?" was "Avoid fat and eat carbohydrates." While the low-fat diet craze reigned supreme throughout the late 1980s and early 1990s, people didn't realize that by eating a low-fat diet, they were actually replacing those fat calories with sugar, also known as refined carbohydrates. Did the low-fat diets make us any thinner? No! In fact, we saw obesity rates skyrocket, leading us to believe that perhaps it isn't fat that makes us fat, and in fact sugar and other carbohydrates may have more to do with it. However, carbohydrates as we know them today were not part of the diet humans ate for millions of years. During the past ten thousand years we have increasingly relied upon cereals and carbohydrates for food, leading to the astronomical rates of obesity, diabetes, and heart disease.

Why do our bodies have such a difficult time adjusting to sugar and other carbohydrate foods? If we take a look at Chapter 2 we see that our bodies are not designed to handle large amounts of sugar and other refined carbohydrates. These foods did not exist when our grandparents and great-grandparents were living. These are modern-day foods that have led to modern-day diseases. In this chapter we will learn to distinguish between the good carbohydrates and the bad carbohydrates, choosing those that our bodies can recognize and that will help prevent and treat insulin resistance.

WHAT ARE CARBOHYDRATES?

Carbohydrates come from a wide array of foods—bread, beans, milk, popcorn, potatoes, cookies, spaghetti, corn, pastries, and others. They also come in a variety of forms. The most common and abundant are sugars, fibers, and starches. The basic building block of a carbohydrate is a sugar molecule, a simple union of carbon, hydrogen, and oxygen. Starches and fibers are essentially chains of sugar molecules. Some contain hundreds of sugars. Some chains are straight, while others branch wildly.

Carbohydrates were once grouped into two main categories. Simple carbohydrates included sugars such as fruit sugar (fructose), corn or grape sugar (dextrose or glucose), and table sugar (sucrose). Complex carbohydrates included everything made of three or more linked sugars and came mainly from fruits, vegetables, and fibrous foods like oatmeal and whole grains. Simple sugars were considered bad and complex carbohydrates good. The picture is much more complicated than that.

The digestive system handles all carbohydrates in much the same way—it breaks them down (or tries to break them down) into single sugar molecules, since only these are small enough to cross into the bloodstream. It also converts most digestible carbohydrates into glucose (also known as blood sugar), because cells are designed to use glucose as a universal energy source.

Fiber is put together in such a way that it can't be broken down into sugar molecules. It passes through the body undigested.

NO CARBOHYDRATES?

The resurgence of the Atkins diet and the rise of the South Beach and other low-carbohydrate diets have put the focus on carbohydrates. While easily digested carbohydrates from white bread, white rice, pastries, and other highly processed foods may contribute to weight gain and interfere with weight loss, that doesn't mean that all carbohydrates are suspect. The Atkins diet treats all carbohydrates as if they are evil, the root of all body fat and excess weight. While some research shows that a low-carbohydrate diet may help people lose weight more quickly than a low-fat diet, no one knows the long-term effects of eating few or no carbohydrates. Regardless of what you have heard about the dangers of carbohydrates, the right carbohydrates are still an important part of a healthy diet.

GOOD CARBS, BETTER CARBS

Just as not all fats are created equal, nor are all carbohydrates. Some kinds promote health, while others, when eaten often and in large quantities, increase insulin resistance, leading to metabolic syndrome, type 2 diabetes, and heart disease. For example, refined sugars and carbohydrates rapidly boost blood sugar levels. To reduce high sugar levels, the pancreas secretes large amounts of insulin, which helps transport the sugar from your food into cells where it is burned for energy (chiefly in muscle cells) or stored as glycogen (in the liver) or fat (in adipose cells). Over time, if you have continually high levels of sugar, insulin levels must remain high to deal with this excess sugar, and elevated insulin levels overwhelm the limited number of insulin cell receptors, stressing them and making them resistant to insulin. You then end up with insulin resistance syndrome or metabolic syndrome.

WHEN SUGAR MANAGEMENT GOES AWRY

Digestible carbohydrates are broken down in the intestine into their simplest form, sugar, which then enters the blood. As the blood sugar level rises, special cells in the pancreas churn out more and more insulin, a hormone that signals cells to absorb blood sugar for energy or storage. As cells absorb blood sugar, the sugar level in the bloodstream falls back to a preset minimum. So does the insulin level.

In some people, this cycle doesn't work properly. Such people have a condition known as insulin resistance, which causes both blood sugar and insulin levels to stay high long after the food has been eaten. Over time, the heavy demands made on the insulin-making cells wear them out, and insulin production slows, then stops. Genes, a sedentary lifestyle, being overweight, and eating foods that cause high spikes in blood sugar can all promote insulin resistance. Data from the Insulin Resistance Atherosclerosis Study suggest that cutting back on refined grains and eating more whole grains in their place can improve insulin sensitivity.

The impact on the body of a carbohydrate can be explained as follows:
Food is eaten
Digestible carbohydrates in food are broken down into glucose
Glucose enters bloodstream (some sugar stored in liver for later access)
Blood sugar rises
Pancreas releases insulin
Glucose leaves bloodstream and enters tissues
Glucose is used as fuel
Glucose supply runs out
Insulin levels drop
Stored sugar in liver is released into bloodstream via glucagon

SUGAR ADDICTS

Sugar was not part of the human diet thousands of years ago. People had almonds and chestnuts; apples and figs and grapes and olives; barley and wheat and rye; berries and melons; milk and honey and a multitude of natural goodness. All of these were brimming with natural sugars, but no refined sugar. Our ancestors used to consume about four pounds of sugar per year. Currently, the average person eats 150 pounds of sugar, which is equivalent to more than half a cup per day. Statistics show that one child in five consumes the recommended minimum of five fruits and vegetables a day, while the top ten sources of carbohydrates in children's diets include soft drinks, cakes, cookies, jam, fruit drinks, and fruit snacks. It's not necessarily all our own fault, though, when you consider the money spent marketing fast foods, convenience foods, and sugary sodas like Coca-Cola and Pepsi. The message of "eat sugar" is everywhere.

Most people are addicted to sugar and grain, and this overconsumption is one of the major health problems facing our nation today. In the late 1970s William Dufty wrote a best-selling book called *Sugar Blues*, warning people of the dangers of sugar. Even thirty-five years ago, he stated, "sugar is the greatest evil that modern industrial civilization has visited upon countries." Although most people do not consider food a drug, sugar, white flour, and refined carbohydrates are akin to drugs as they are addictive substances that affect brain neurotransmitters similar to those produced by alcohol. The taste for sweets leads to a craving for more sugar, just the way other drugs create cravings. The human body cannot handle refined sugar. Not only does this excessive consumption of sugar lead to insulin resistance, metabolic syndrome, and increased risk of developing type 2 diabetes, but excess sugar in the bloodstream stimulates the generation of free radicals. In blood vessels, free radical damage causes an accumulation of plaque that can lead to blocked arteries and cardiovascular disease.

ASPARTAME POISONING

Many of you have started to hear and learn about the dangers of sugar, so in an effort to preserve your health, you have made the switch to aspartame, Sucralose, and Acesulfame-K. But are these any healthier than good old table sugar, sucrose? No. These are artificial chemical sweeteners with questionable safety records.

Although aspartame (the artificial sweetener known as NutraSweet) is approved by the Food and Drug Administration (FDA), composed of natural ingredients, and found in literally thousands of products, including those intended for dieters and diabetics, it isn't necessarily safe.

So why haven't we all heard about the dangers of aspartame? Partly because the diet industry is worth trillions of dollars, and the manufacturers of diet products want to protect their profits by hiding the truth about aspartame's dangers. The number of complaints to the FDA is reaching astronomical numbers; in fact, one report stated 85% of all complaints registered to the FDA are for adverse reactions to aspartame, including five reported deaths.

What makes aspartame so dangerous? What seems to be a relatively simple chemical composition is really dangerous. Aspartame is made of two amino acids, aspartic acid and phenylalanine, which are fused together by a third component, methanol. When methanol is released it becomes a poisonous free radical that damages cells and is a leading contributor to many diseases. Methanol is a known carcinogen, and has been known to cause birth defects.

Although phenylalanine is an essential amino acid, in isolated form it can have dangerous side effects, especially to those sensitive to the amino acid and to those who are phenylketonuric. It can be harmful to diabetics and may cause altered brain function and behavior changes. Many people have reported the following side effects from aspartame: fibromyalgia, multiple sclerosis symptoms, dizziness, headaches, and menstrual problems.

Avoiding Hidden Aspartame

Please check labels carefully and compare contents to the list of "sweeteners to avoid" in Table 4.1. Aspartame and many other artificial sweeteners can be found in the following products: soft drinks, over-the-counter drugs and prescription drugs, yogurt, instant breakfasts, candy, breath mints, cereals, sugar-free chewing gum, cocoa mixes, coffee beverages, gelatin desserts, juice beverages, tabletop sweeteners, topping mixes, and many more.

Many people find it much easier to avoid toxic sweeteners by shopping at health food stores when possible. Many health food stores have banned artificial sweeteners for obvious reasons, but it is still important to check labels.

THE RIGHT SWEETENERS: XYLITOL AND STEVIA

You are probably wondering what kind of sweetener/sugar you should be using, after reading about the dangers of aspartame. I have included a chart listing healthy and unhealthy sweeteners, but I will expand on my two preferences—xylitol and stevia.

Table 4.1: Which Sweeteners to Use and Which to Avoid

Sweeteners to Use	Sweeteners to Avoid
Stevia*	Aspartame (NutraSweet, Equal, Canderel)
Honey	Neotame
Rice syrup	Sucralose (Splenda)
Xylitol	Acesulfame-K (Sunette, Sweet & Safe, Sweet One)
Licorice Root (small amounts)	Cyclamates
Fructooligosaccharides	Saccharin
Agave nectar and syrup*	Refined Sugar
Fruit Juice	High Fructose Sweeteners
Evaporated Cane Juice	Brown Sugar
Amasake	Corn Syrup
Other Sugar Alcohols **	Dextrose
Sweet Fiber ®*	
* Safe for Diabetics	
** Use in Small Amounts	

Herbal Stevia

Stevia Rebaudiana (a herb from Brazil and Paraguay) is an all-natural herbal sweetener that has virtually no calories and no glycemic effect, so it doesn't spike blood sugar levels. It's my top choice for natural sweeteners. If you've ever tasted it, you know it's extremely sweet, in fact two or three hundred times sweeter than sugar, meaning only very small amounts need to be used. The glycosides in its leaves, which include up to ten percent Stevioside, account for its incredible sweetness. It is available in many forms—tablets, powders, and liquid drops—and can be used in baking, coffee, tea, and so on.

Xylitol

Xylitol, discovered by Finnish scientists, is a high-grade sweetener that comes from birch bark. It has a very low glycemic index, even though it is a sugar alcohol. It is also anti-bacterial and has actually been shown to prevent dental cavities. Xylitol has been used in products such as nasal wash, toothpaste, and mouthwash.

Some people experience minor gastrointestinal disturbances from using sugar alcohols, especially maltitol and sorbitol. Xylitol is considered a five-carbon sugar, whereas sugar and sorbitol are six-carbon sugars. The five-carbon sugars are antimicrobial, preventing the growth of bacteria. The six-carbon sugars feed dangerous bacteria and fungi, which then may cause stomach upset. As well, our bodies produce xylitol and the enzymes required to break it down, so our bodies are well equipped to deal with xylitol as a natural sweetener.

Xylitol looks, feels, and tastes exactly like sugar, and leaves no unpleasant aftertaste. It is available in many forms. It can replace sugar in cooking, baking, or as a sweetener for beverages.

CARBOHYDRATES AND THE GLYCEMIC INDEX

A new system for classifying carbohydrates calls into question many of the old assumptions about how carbohydrates affect health. This new system, known as the glycemic index, measures how fast blood sugar rises after you eat a food that contains carbohydrates.

White sugar is converted almost immediately to blood sugar, causing blood sugar levels to spike rapidly. It's classified as having a high glycemic index. Brown rice, in contrast, is digested more slowly, causing a lower and more gentle change in blood sugar. It has a low glycemic index.

The most comprehensive list of the glycemic index of foods was published in the July 2002 issue of the *American Journal of Clinical Nutrition*. A version of the glycemic index is in the Appendix. For further information on the glycemic index and load of foods, you can visit an online resource at www.mendosa.com.

The best food choices are in the low-glycemic group, rated 55 or less. Your goal is to consume the low-glycemic foods, which will cause the least amount of insulin production, to avoid overwhelming your insulin receptor site and causing insulin resistance. Foods with a low glycemic index can help control your blood glucose levels, cholesterol levels, and appetite, and can lower your risk of developing insulin resistance, metabolic syndrome, type 2 diabetes, and heart disease. High-glycemic index foods, which trigger excessive insulin, are also associated with an increase in fat storage. Lowering insulin levels is not only a key ingredient in weight loss and preventing meta-bolic syndrome, but also the secret to long-term health.

Figure 4.1: The Two-Hour Blood Sugar Response
of a High-GI Food vs. a Low-GI Food

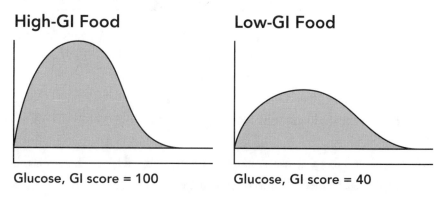

High-GI Food

Low-GI Food

Glucose, GI score = 100   Glucose, GI score = 40

Glycemic index values for different foods are calculated by comparing mea-surements of their effects on blood glucose at an equal carbohydrate portion of a reference food. The current scientific validated methods use glucose as the reference. Glucose has a glycemic index value of 100.

Separating the Whole Grain from the Chaff
Food companies make it more difficult than it should be to spot a whole-grain food. Aware that consumers are interested in whole-grain products, companies often make foods sound like they're whole grain and healthy when they aren't.

That means you must read food labels carefully. True whole-grain products list as the main ingredient whole wheat, whole oats, whole rye, or some other whole-grain cereal. If the label says "made with wheat flour" it may be an intact grain product or it may just be an advertising gimmick, since even highly processed cake flour is made with wheat flour. Breakfast cereals made from whole grains will usually say so in bold letters. Foods that contain 51% or more of whole grains by weight may also carry a government-approved message linking their consumption to a decrease in heart disease and cancer risk. Among the commercially available cereals, good whole-grain choices include shredded wheat products, Cheerios, Wheaties, and Total, and of course All Bran, Bran Buds, and other bran cereals, which can be used as a topping on all cereals. Commercially available whole-wheat breads may be harder to identify because even the most healthy-sounding breads may be made from refined flours instead of whole grains. In other words that 12-grain bread that sounds so good for you could be made entirely with refined flours. If you look at the label and you don't see the word "whole," then chances are the bread is made from refined grains. If you see the word "enriched" instead of "whole," that usually means the grain has been refined.

One of the most important factors that determine a food's glycemic index is how highly processed its carbohydrates are. Processing carbohydrates removes the fiber-rich outer bran and the vitamin- and mineral-rich inner germ, leaving mostly the starchy endosperm. Other factors also influence how quickly the carbohydrates in food raise blood sugar, including:

- *Fiber content:* Fiber shields the starchy carbohydrates in food. This slows the release of sugar molecules into the bloodstream.
- *Ripeness:* Ripe fruits and vegetables tend to have more sugar than unripe ones and so tend to have a higher glycemic index.
- *Types of starch:* Starch comes in many different configurations. Some starches are easier to break into sugar molecules than others. The starch in potatoes, for example, is digested and absorbed into the bloodstream relatively quickly.
- *Food preparation:* How the food is prepared can affect the glycemic response. For example, pasta that is cooked al dente—or firm—has a lower glycemic response than pasta that is overcooked.
- *Fat content:* The more fat a food contains, the slower its carbohydrates are converted into sugar and absorbed into the bloodstream.
- *Physical form:* Finely ground grain is more rapidly digested and so has a higher glycemic index than more coarsely ground grain.

All these elements lead to sometimes counterintuitive results. Some foods that contain complex carbohydrates, such as potatoes, quickly raise blood sugar levels, while some foods that contain simple carbohydrates, such as whole fruit, raise blood sugar levels more slowly.

GLYCEMIC LOAD

There is one thing that a food's glycemic index does not tell us: the relative amount of carbohydrate in a given food. Take watermelon as an example: the sweet-tasting fruit has a high glycemic index, but a slice of watermelon has only a small amount of carbohydrate per serving (as the name implies, watermelon is made up of mostly water). Looking at the glycemic index alone may not tell us everything that we need to know about a food's impact on blood sugar levels. Researchers have developed a new way of classifying foods that takes into account both the amount of carbohydrate in the food and the impact of that carbohydrate on blood sugar levels. This measure is called the glycemic load. A food's glycemic load is determined by multiplying its glycemic index by the amount of carbohydrate it contains (carbohydrate minus fiber) and dividing by 100. You should aim for a daily glycemic load of <100. A high glycemic load is >120. Glycemic Load = (GI Value x Carbohydrate per Serving) /100.

Table 4.2: Carbohydrates and the Glycemic Load*

Low Glycemic Load = 10 or Less	Medium Glycemic Load = 11-19	High Glycemic Load = 20 or More
High fiber fruits and vegetables, not including potatoes	Pearled Barley, 1 cup cooked	Baked Potato
Bran Cereals (1 oz)	Brown Rice, 3/4 cup, cooked	French Fries
Many legumes, including chickpeas, kidney beans, black beans, lentils, pinto beans (5 oz cooked, approx 3/4 cup)	Oatmeal, 1 cup, cooked	Refined Cereals, 1 oz or 30 g
	Bulgur, 3/4 cup cooked	Sugar-sweetened beverages, 12 oz
	Rice cakes, 3 cakes	Jelly beans, 10 large
	Whole-grain breads, 1 slice	Candy bars, 1 to 2 oz bar or 3 mini bars
	Whole-grain pasta, 1 1/4 cup cooked	Couscous, 1 cup, cooked

Continued

Low Glycemic Load = 10 or Less	Medium Glycemic Load = 11-19	High Glycemic Load = 20 or More
	No sugar added fruit juice, 8 oz	Cranberry cocktail, 8 oz
		White pasta, 1 cup, cooked

*Glycemic load categorization adapted from Foster-Powell K, Holt SH, Brand-Miller JC. International table of glycemic index and glycemic load values: 2002. *Am J Clin Nutr* 2002; 76:5-56.

Although the fine points of the glycemic index and glycemic load may seem complicated, the basic message is simple: whenever possible, replace highly processed grains, cereals, and sugars with minimally processed whole-grain products. This will bring us back to the basics of eating, yet still take into account the changes in our lifestyle and the modern-day foods we have available to us.

GETTING STARTED ON THE LOW-GI EATING PLAN

Although this new way of eating carbohydrates can seem daunting, it doesn't have to be. Follow these simple tips to start eating according to the glycemic index.

- Start the day with whole grains. If you're partial to hot cereals, try old-fashioned or steel-cut oats, or barley.
- Use whole-grain breads for lunch or snacks. Check the label to make sure that whole wheat or other whole grain is the first ingredient listed.
- Try new foods that have a low GI. Experiment with beans, legumes, and lentils by including them in dishes such as chili, soups, and salad.
- If you choose a high-GI food, combine it with a low-GI food for an overall medium-GI meal. For example, a high-GI cereal topped with a spoonful of All Bran (low GI) and some strawberries (low GI).
- Limit the amount of processed, refined, starchy foods, as they tend to be lower in fiber and other nutrients and have a higher GI.
- Unlimited vegetables—you can eat most vegetables without thinking about their glycemic index. Most are so low in carbohydrate that they have no

measurable effect on blood sugar levels. Avoid the higher GI foods mentioned above, for example, potato, corn, and peas. Corn and sweet potato are lower GI than peas and potato. Veggies such as tomatoes, lettuce, cucumbers, peppers, and onions can be considered "free foods" as even in large amounts they have no effect on blood sugar levels.

• You may be wondering why there are no GI values for meat, nuts, and most "fat" foods like avocadoes. These foods contain very little or no carbohydrate, so you can consider their glycemic index as 0.

WHOLE GRAINS REDUCE METABOLIC SYNDROME

In its 2005 Dietary Guidelines, the United States Department of Agriculture recommends at least three ounces of whole-grain cereals, crackers, breads, pasta, or rice daily. The reason? Whole grains are high in fiber, vitamins, minerals, and phytochemicals (plant compounds that help reduce the risk of several chronic diseases and ailments), and they increase the soluble and insoluble fiber intake, which is often sorely lacking in North American diets. On average, North Americans consume only 0.9 to 1.1 servings of whole grains per day. Equally dismaying is the inadequate total daily consumption of fiber, which is around 12 to 18 grams per day, a far cry from the recommended 25 to 38 grams per day.

Other large cohort studies have found similar results. In a study in 2004 published in *Diabetes Care*, the researchers analyzed data from 2,834 subjects at the fifth examination (1991 to 1995) of the Framingham Offspring Study. Metabolic syndrome was defined using the National Cholesterol Education Program Criteria (see Chapter 1). After adjusting for potential confounding variables, intakes of total dietary fiber, cereal fiber, fruit fiber, and whole grains were inversely associated with insulin resistance, whereas a high glycemic index and glycemic load were positively associated with the disorder. The prevalence of the metabolic syndrome was significantly lower among those in the highest quintile of cereal-fiber and whole-grain intakes compared to those in the lowest quintile. The researchers reported that, because both a high cereal fiber content and a lower glycemic index are attributes of whole-grain foods, recommendations to increase whole-grain intake may reduce the risk of developing the metabolic syndrome.

A study published in the *American Journal of Clinical Nutrition* in November 2003 found that higher whole-grain intake is associated with increased insulin sensitivity. An increased intake of whole-grain foods has been related to a reduced risk of developing diabetes and heart disease. One underlying pathway for this connection may be increased insulin sensitivity. The investigators in this study evaluated data from the Insulin Resistance Atherosclerosis Study (IRAS). They found that those subjects who increased their intake of whole grains had increased insulin sensitivity after adjusting for demographics, total energy intake and expenditure, smoking, and family history of diabetes. Upon analysis of the nutritional component of their food, they also found the presence of fiber and magnesium in whole-grain products might explain a significant amount of the association to insulin sensitivity. The investigators of the study concluded that as insulin sensitivity is one of the main predictors of diabetes, their findings confirm the protective effects of whole grains on the risk of developing diabetes.

A BOWLFUL OF CEREAL A DAY KEEPS THE DOCTOR AWAY

Eating a bowlful of high-fiber cereal may help prevent type 2 diabetes and other health problems in people at risk for developing the disease. In a study published in *Diabetes Care*, the researchers showed that eating a high-fiber cereal lowered insulin production and reduced blood glucose levels in men with elevated insulin levels, a precursor to metabolic syndrome. People with high insulin levels are in danger of developing type 2 diabetes because the cells in their bodies are resistant to the effects of insulin and cannot process sugar properly. This causes the pancreas to produce more insulin in order to compensate. High insulin levels and insulin resistance are also associated with an increased risk of heart disease. By lowering the rise in insulin and

blood sugar levels that normally follows eating a meal high in carbohydrates, researchers say that people at risk for developing diabetes may be able to ward off the disease and its complications.

The researchers compared the effects of eating a high- or low-fiber ready-to-eat breakfast cereal in seventy-seven men without diabetes. Forty-two men had elevated insulin levels. The men in the high-fiber cereal group ate 1.3 cups of cereal—Fiber One from General Mills—which provided nearly 36 grams of fiber. The low-fiber cereal group ate Country Corn Flakes from General Mills, which had less than 1 gram of fiber in the 1-cup serving size.

The study showed that blood sugar levels were significantly lower in all the men after eating the high-fiber cereal than after eating the low-fiber cereal. In addition, insulin production was significantly lower after eating the high-fiber cereal than after eating the low-fiber cereal. In addition, in men with high insulin levels, insulin production was significantly lower after they ate the high-fiber cereal than after they ate the low-fiber cereal.

FIX IT WITH FIBER: THE IMPORTANCE OF DIETARY FIBER

More than sixty years ago, scientists began to study the effects of food fiber on human health. At first, scientists believed that fiber had little to no nutritional value and was unimportant in any food or diet. During the grain milling process, bran (which is all fiber) was removed, leaving behind white, starchy flour, stripped of fiber and other essential nutrients. The milling helped improve the functionality and appearance of the flour, and bakers found that this refined flour worked better for making bread and other baked products, but they didn't realize the detrimental health effects that the lack of fiber would have on our health.

Research continued to evolve in this area, and scientists such as Dr. Dennis Burkitt began looking at the diets of people living in countries with high-fiber diets. The researchers found that these people typically did not experience constipation and other types of gastrointestinal diseases, heart disease, obesity, and type 2 diabetes, which were rampant in the Western populations who consumed diets high in processed and convenience foods, inadequate amounts of fruits and vegetables, and little or no fiber. A steady diet of refined carbohydrates depletes the body of essential nutrients and leaves it unable to digest these carbohydrates, increasing the body's toxic load. Scientific opinions have definitely evolved regarding fiber's role. Although fiber does not have any nutritional value as it passes through the bowels undigested, it has many vital functions in the body. From these data, the research and medical community began to understand the importance of fiber in the diet.

Today, we still live in a fiber-deficient society. The majority of North Americans consume only one quarter to one-half of the Institute of Medicine's 2002 recommended fiber levels of 38 grams per day for men and 25 grams per day for women. The average daily fiber intake is only 12 grams for women and 18 grams for men.

TYPES OF FIBER

There are two main types of fiber that are important for health: soluble and insoluble. Soluble fiber is found in flax seed, oats, barley, and legumes and in smaller amounts in fruits and vegetables. Soluble fiber forms a gelatin-like substance and increases the water content of the stool. Soluble fiber acts like a sponge, binding excess toxins, blood cholesterol, and blood sugar, and is an important nutrient for the dietary management of high cholesterol and diabetes. For example, a research study published in the British Journal of Nutrition confirmed the positive effects on persons consuming 40 grams of ground flax seeds daily during a four-week study. The blood glucose levels were reduced by 27%, while cholesterol levels were reduced by 7%.

Insoluble fiber is found in flax seeds, wheat, bran and whole grains, and in smaller amounts in fruits and vegetables. Insoluble fiber sweeps the colon, increases stool size, and helps relieve constipation and gas. Research also shows that consuming sufficient amounts of insoluble fiber plays an important role in satiety (feeling of fullness), and may help people lose weight. Obesity is less prevalent in populations that consume a high-fiber diet.

Table 4.3: Sources of Fiber

Soluble Fiber	Insoluble Fiber
Oatmeal	Whole grains, such as whole wheat breads, barley, couscous, brown rice, and bulgur
Oat bran	Whole-grain breakfast cereals
Nuts and seeds	Wheat bran
Legumes such as dried peas, beans, and lentils	Seeds
Apples	Carrots
Pears	Cucumbers
Strawberries	Zucchini
Blueberries	Celery
	Tomatoes

There are numerous benefits to consuming fiber. A high-fiber diet will promote increased chewing and slower eating, delay gastric emptying (keeping you feeling full for up to four hours after a meal), stabilize blood sugar levels, absorb toxins, reduce cholesterol in your blood, increase stool size, and reduce your overall risk of chronic disease.

FIBER AND WEIGHT CONTROL

A new study published in the *Journal of the American Dietetic Association* in September 2005 confirmed that women who want to lose weight should place emphasis on dietary fiber rather than on low-carb, low-fat, and high-protein diets. The study was based on the 4,539 people who participated in the Continuing Survey of Food Intakes between 1994 and 1996. The survey found that only five percent reported an adequate intake of fiber. It was found that for women, a low-fiber, high-fat diet increased the risk of being overweight or obese. Beyond weight control, the researchers concluded that a fiber-rich diet provides a wide range of health benefits for both men and women, such as lower blood cholesterol levels, a reduced risk of digestive diseases, and a possible reduction in the risk of heart disease. In the light of these benefits the researchers concluded that increased fiber consumption should be promoted to men and women.

FIBER AND METABOLIC SYNDROME

Insufficient fiber intake has been linked with metabolic syndrome. Consuming a whole-grain-rich diet is associated with reducing the risk of metabolic syndrome, type 2 diabetes, and heart disease, according to a recent study performed by researchers at Tufts University. The researchers found that people who ate more whole-grains and cereal fiber and followed diets with lower glycemic index foods showed better insulin sensitivity and were less likely to be affected by insulin resistance or metabolic syndrome. Those who ate three or more servings of whole-grain foods daily were at the lowest risk for metabolic syndrome.

FIBER AND HEART DISEASE

In North America, coronary heart disease is a leading cause of death for both men and women. This disease is characterized by a buildup of cholesterol-filled plaque in the coronary arteries, which feed the heart. This buildup causes the arteries to become hard and narrow, a process referred to as atherosclerosis. Total blockage of a coronary artery produces a heart attack.

High intake of dietary fiber has been linked to a lower risk of heart disease in a number of large studies that followed people for many years. In a Harvard study of more than 40,000 male health professionals, researchers found that a high total dietary fiber intake was linked to a forty percent lower risk of coronary heart disease, compared to a low fiber intake. Cereal fiber, the fiber found in grains, seemed particularly beneficial. A related study of Harvard female nurses produced similar findings.

FIBER AND TYPE 2 DIABETES

When it comes to factors that increase the risk of developing diabetes, a diet low in cereal fiber and rich in high-glycemic foods seems particularly bad. The Harvard studies mentioned in the heart disease section found that this sort of diet more than doubled the risk of type 2 diabetes when compared to a diet high in cereal fiber and low in high-glycemic index foods.

Viscofiber, a New Fiber Ingredient

Research into soluble fiber components of dietary fiber has led to the discovery of fractions of oat soluble fiber—beta glucans—that have been shown to effectively lower blood cholesterol, reduce postprandial blood glucose, induce satiety, and suppress appetite.

Viscofiber is a natural superior ingredient with an enhanced concentration of soluble fiber (12 times more than oat bran). Viscofiber delivers the highest viscosity available. It contains more than 50% B-glucans from oats. The importance of viscosity has been accepted by the FDA and well documented by leading fiber scientists as the major property responsible for the physiological effects of consuming viscous soluble fiber, such as lowering cholesterol and glucose levels. Viscofiber has been shown to be twenty to thirty times more viscous than the next leading B-glucan concentrate.

B-glucan is found in the cell walls of grains, and the process used to make Viscofiber allows the structure of the natural grain to remain relatively unchanged, preserving the original high viscosity of B-glucan. Just a few grams of this novel ingredient offer the multiple heart health advantages of consuming four bowls of oatmeal.

The mechanism of how B-glucan works in the body is well understood and attributed to viscous soluble fiber, followed by insoluble fibers and accompanying substances. Viscofiber has many unique characteristics (described below) that together result in multiple heart health benefits.

Glycemic Response: Viscofiber has been clinically studied for its effects on glycemic response and cholesterol response. The high viscosity associated with Viscofiber increases the duration of intestinal transit and results in delaying digestion of available carbohydrates, leading to a reduction of glycemic response. Multiple clinical trials using Viscofiber have demonstrated a dose response effect, meaning the more you consume, the better the results for improving glucose and insulin levels.

Cholesterol Response: When Viscofiber is eaten, the oat soluble fiber forms a gel in the small intestine that surrounds bile acids and prevents them from being reabsorbed through the walls of the small intestine and recycled to the liver. Consequently, the bile acids are trapped by the gel and are excreted from the body by forcing the liver to take cholesterol out of the blood to replace the bile acids that have been excreted. The result is reduced total and LDL cholesterol.

Research done in 2004 at St. Michael's Hospital at the University of Toronto by Dr. Vladimir Vuksan evaluated the effects of Viscofiber on glycemic response. Eight grams of beta glucan taken in the form of a beverage resulted in a 38% reduction in after-meal glucose, a 56% reduction in insulin secretion, and a 65% improvement in insulin sensitivity. Additionally increasing doses of Viscofiber correspond to an even greater reduction in insulin and glycemic response. No other B-glucan concentrate available is like Viscofiber! Viscofiber is a powerful fiber ingredient with a significant impact on the prevention of insulin resistance and metabolic syndrome.

WHAT YOU HAVE LEARNED IN THIS CHAPTER

- Not all carbohydrates are created equally. There are sugars, fibers, and complex carbohydrates found in legumes and whole grains. We need to avoid sugar and focus our diet on fiber and complex carbohydrates.
- Carbohydrates can be classified based on their glycemic index (GI), which measures how quickly the food will be turned into sugar and enter our bloodstream, and the glycemic load (GL), which tells us the amount of carbohydrate in a given food. Choose low-GI and low-GL foods as your carbohydrate sources.
- Emphasize dietary fiber from fruits, vegetables, and whole grains. New soluble fiber ingredients are available, for example Viscofiber, which has been clinically studied. The study showed that it lowers glycemic response and improve insulin sensitivity.

In the next chapter we will look at the importance of protein in our diet for preventing insulin resistance and metabolic syndrome.

Chapter 5

PROTEIN POWER

Every decade seems to have its hot nutrient. The 80s had carbs, the 90s were the fat decade. Now the hot nutrient is protein. There's the protein diet, the high-protein diet, and the even-higher-protein diet. But how much protein do we really require? What foods contain it? Which protein is best? And will protein help prevent insulin resistance and diabetes?

The concept of a high-protein, low-carbohydrate diet is not new. In fact most anthropological evidence suggests our stone-age ancestors were hunter-gatherers who subsisted on a diet rich in meats, wild green plants, berries, and shrub fruits. Throughout evolution our diet has undergone significant changes, but many experts feel that our bodies are still best suited to a high-protein, low-carbohydrate diet.

Diets such as the Dr. Atkins diet promote high protein/low carbohydrate eating, much like the diet believed to be consumed by our ancestors during the Paleolithic period. However, the long-term consequences of a high-protein diet are not known. Even though protein foods do not cause insulin to spike, high-protein, low-carbohydrate diets are not necessarily the solution for people who are insulin resistant because the types of protein foods advocated in this diet are also high in fat, especially saturated fat, the type that can promote insulin resistance.

Restricting carbohydrates can be very dangerous. As we discussed in Chapter 4, not all carbohydrates are created equally, and we need to focus on the low-glycemic carbohydrates and dietary fiber that are very important for preventing insulin resistance. As well, the proteins our ancestors consumed were very different from the proteins of today, because of changes in the way we feed our livestock—the change from grass-fed to grain-fed has resulted in meat that is of poorer quality and higher in the pro-inflammatory types of fat that are linked to insulin resistance.

This is why we need to be very careful to choose high-quality protein. I am not advocating a high-protein diet, which is also typically high in fat, but I am suggesting that we consume a high-quality protein source at each meal and with each snack, which we will talk about later on. Balancing protein with carbohydrates and fat is the key to preventing and managing insulin resistance. If we remember what we discussed in the last two chapters, we need to:

- Decrease saturated and trans fats.
- Incorporate more essential fatty acids from nuts, seeds, fatty fish, and green leafy vegetables, as well as the healthy omega-9 fats from olive oil and avocadoes.
- Decrease consumption of refined carbohydrates, including white sugar, white rice, and white pasta.
- Increase consumption of fibrous, low-glycemic foods.
- Choose high-quality proteins, and balance protein foods at snack time and mealtime.

WHAT IS PROTEIN?

Proteins are essential components of the body and are required for its structure and proper function. Proteins function as enzymes, hormones, and antibodies, as well as transport and structural components. Proteins comprise building blocks called amino acids. Of the twenty amino acids, the body makes twelve, which are called nonessential. The other eight are the essential amino acids, which, like essential fatty acids, must be supplied by the diet. These include leucine, isoleucine, valine, threonine, methionine, phenylalanine, tryptophan, and lysine.

DIETARY SOURCES OF PROTEIN

Most foods contain at least some protein. Good sources of protein include lean meat, fish, and poultry, nuts and seeds, pulses (edible seeds of certain pod-bearing plants, such as beans and peas), soy products (tofu, soy milk), cereals (wheat, oats, and rice), eggs, and some dairy products (milk, cheese, and yogurt).

Different foods contain different proteins, each with its own unique amino acid composition. The proportions of essential amino acids in foods may differ from the proportions needed by the body to make proteins. The proportion of each of the essential amino acids in foods containing protein determines the quality of that protein. A dietary protein that contains all the essential amino acids in the proportions required by the body is said to be a high-quality protein. If the protein is low in one or more of the essential amino acids, the protein is of lower quality.

Protein quality is usually defined according to the amino acid pattern of egg protein, which is regarded as the ideal. So it is not surprising that animal proteins, such as meat, milk, and cheese, tend to be of a higher quality than plant proteins. This is why plant proteins are sometimes referred to as low-quality proteins. Many plant proteins are low in one of the essential amino acids. For instance, grains tend to be short of lysine, while pulses are short of methionine.

This does not mean that vegetarians go short on essential amino acids. Combining plant proteins, like corn (limited in lysine) with beans (limited in methionine), leads to a high-quality protein combination that is just as good as, and in some cases better than, protein from animal foods. Beans on toast, cheese or a peanut butter sandwich, muesli with milk, and rice with peas or beans are all common examples of protein complementing. Soy is a high-quality protein on its own that is equal to meat protein.

Table 5.1: Recommended Protein Sources

Good Sources		Fair Sources
Chickpeas	Eggs	Brown rice
Baked beans	Tuna fish packed in water	Broccoli
Tofu	Salmon packed in water	Corn
Cow's milk	Peanut butter (natural, no trans fats)	Bulgur
Soy milk	Cottage cheese	
Lentils	Lean cuts of meat, fish, poultry	
Muesli	Natural yogurt	
Peanuts	Multigrain cereal, for example Red River	
Hard cheese	Whey protein powder	

Combining proteins with low-glycemic carbohydrates is essential to help balance the effects on blood glucose and insulin levels. It also ensures a feeling of fullness and helps in maintaining muscle. Protein is needed to build the body (hair, nails, bone matrix, cell membranes, enzymes). From a weight-control perspective, protein helps curb the appetite. Adequate protein intake also means a person is eating less fat and carbohydrate.

If we don't eat enough protein, our bodies can't perform all the functions for which protein is required. Over time, we may feel tired and sluggish, and be more susceptible to illness. We fail to build muscle, which can lead to insulin resistance and weight gain.

BALANCING PROTEIN

So how much protein does one really need to consume? My preference is to consume a protein food every time I eat.

The average recommended daily requirement for protein for adults is 50 grams for females and 70 grams for males. A person who is very physically active and/or trying to lose weight may want to increase the consumption of protein.

Registered dietitian Leslie Beck, author of *The Complete Idiot's Guide to Total Nutrition for Canadians*, gives the following recommendations based on activity levels.

Exercise Category	Recommended Daily Protein Intake (Grams per pound of body weight)
Sedentary	0.36
Moderate	0.36–0.5
Endurance	0.5–0.8
Teenage	0.6–0.9

However, I don't recommend just any protein from animal foods, as some contain significantly higher levels of saturated fat, one of the main culprits in insulin resistance. Overall, aim for 15 to 20% of calories from protein, 45 to 50% from fibrous, low-glycemic index carbohydrates, and no more than 25 to 30% from fat, with a focus on the mono and polyunsaturated fats.

You are probably wondering how to determine how much protein you are eating at each meal. Three to seven servings (see Chapter 10, Table 10.3 for information on serving sizes) of meat, dairy, fish, and meat alternatives like legumes and beans is a good start. In practical terms, this means consuming a protein at each meal and with each snack. I am a firm believer in eating five to six small meals a day. This helps keep your blood sugar levels stable, helps prevent insulin resistance, keeps you feeling full and satisfied throughout the day, and keeps your metabolism revved up.

For example, you could drink two whey protein shakes per day and also eat three small meals. Drink one protein shake (containing 20 to 25 grams of whey protein) mid-morning and another an hour before dinner. The protein shakes will control your appetite at common craving times.

High-quality whey protein has been shown in the scientific data to promote weight loss and insulin sensitivity, and is a great way to meet your protein requirements. By consuming a protein shake one or two times per day you are able to meet your protein requirements as well as many other nutrient requirements. I love making power protein smoothies in the morning in my blender. Drinking a protein shake is a great way to start the day, and provides all the nutrients you need to lose weight. See my recipe for Flax Berry Blast on page 217 in Chapter 13.

You can also mix whey protein powder with water or a milk beverage for an easy afternoon snack. Whey protein powder can be mixed into almost any food.

Beverages
- Water
- Milk beverage
- Sports drinks (check the sugar content, as some contain very high levels of sugar)
- Fruit or vegetable juice

Cold Foods
- Applesauce
- Cold cereal
- Cottage cheese
- Peanut butter/almond butter
- Yogurt

Hot Foods
- Hot cereal
- Old-fashioned oats
- Chili
- Soup
- Pasta sauce
- Ground meat

Overall, protein should be incorporated into each meal and snack to balance blood sugar levels.

PROTEIN KEEPS YOU FULL

When people follow a diet such as Atkins, even if they know it may not be the healthiest diet, their comment is, "It works." If you are consuming more fat, why does this carbohydrate-restricted diet help you lose weight? One of the reasons may be the increased intake of protein. In a study published in the *American Journal of Clinical Nutrition*, nineteen middle-age overweight men and women were studied while they consumed a diet that provided various ratios of protein, fat, and carbohydrates. During the first two weeks, they followed diets that were designed to maintain body weight and that contained 15% of calories as protein, 35% as fat, and 50% as carbohydrate. In the next two weeks, the composition of the diet was adjusted to provide 30% of calories as protein, 20% as fat, and the same 50% as carbohydrate. The total amount of calories remained unchanged. Over the final twelve weeks, the subjects were instructed to eat as much as they wished of the same high-protein protocol. Measurements at the start of each dietary period and at the end of the study included body weight and composition, metabolic rates, insulin levels, and the appetite-regulating hormones ghrelin (the hormones responsible for satiety) and leptin (the hormone responsible for hunger). Findings included unchanged weight during the first two weeks and weight-maintenance periods of prescribed total calories. However, during the twelve-week phase of unrestricted total calorie intake with the high-protein, low-fat diet, there was an average decrease of 450 calories per day and a 5 kg (11 pound) weight loss. These findings were accompanied by an increased sense of fullness; significantly decreased levels of leptin, and increased levels of ghrelin. The authors conclude that the high-protein diet increased brain sensitivity to the hormonal regulation of appetite without affecting energy expenditure. The overall message is to emphasize complex carbohydrates such as the low-glycemic carbohydrates (including increased dietary fiber), high protein, and low saturated fats to achieve maximal health benefits.

THE WHEY IT IS

Many of you will have difficulty achieving the recommended levels of high-quality protein through diet alone. Not that meeting the protein requirements is difficult, because in fact most North Americans get plenty of protein. The problem is that protein-laden foods are associated with high levels of fat and cholesterol. One of the nutrition products I include in my personal nutrition regime is whey protein. Supplemental whey protein ensures that your protein needs can be met in the highest quality way. Whey protein is a naturally complete protein, meaning that it contains all the essential amino acids required in the daily diet. It has the ideal combination of amino acids to help improve body composition and enhance athletic performance.

Branched-Chain Amino Acids

Whey protein is a rich source of branched-chain amino acids (BCAAs); it contains the highest known levels found in any natural food source. BCAAs include leucine, isoleucine, and valine, and are important for athletes, because, unlike the other essential amino acids, they are metabolized directly into muscle tissue and are the first ones used during exercise and resistance training. Whey protein is also an excellent source of the essential amino acid leucine. Leucine plays a key role in promoting muscle protein synthesis and muscle growth. Research has shown that individuals who exercise benefit from diets high in leucine and have more lean muscle tissue and less body fat than individuals whose diet contains lower levels of leucine. Whey protein isolate has about 50% more leucine than soy protein isolate.

Whey protein is a soluble, easy to digest protein and is efficiently absorbed into the body. It is a fast protein due to its ability to quickly provide nourishment to the muscles.

Whey to Weight Loss

A diet based on increased but not excessive levels of protein has been shown in a number of studies to give an added boost to dieters by helping them increase weight loss, increase loss of body fat, and reduce the loss of muscle tissue. But how can people easily add more protein to their diets without overdoing it? Whey protein is a great option. The body requires more energy to digest protein than other foods, so we burn more calories after a protein meal. Whey protein is pure protein with little to no fat or carbohydrates. It is a perfect complement to a low-glycemic index diet plan. Recent studies have highlighted the role of the essential amino acid leucine in improving body composition. High-quality whey protein is rich in leucine, which helps preserve lean muscle tissue while promoting fat loss. Whey protein contains more leucine than milk protein, egg protein, and soy protein.

Protein helps stabilize blood glucose levels by slowing the absorption of glucose into the bloodstream. This in turn reduces hunger by lowering insulin levels and making it easier for the body to burn fat. Whey protein contains components that help stimulate the release of two appetite-suppressing hormones: cholecystokinin (CCK) and glucagon-like-peptide(GLP-1). In support of this, a new study found that whey protein had a greater impact on satiety than casein, the other protein in milk.

A six-month study of sixty-five overweight and obese people, published in 1999 in the *International Journal of Obesity*, compared two low-calorie diets: one with twelve percent of calories from protein and one with twenty-five percent of calories from protein. Those who ate more protein lost more weight, irrespective of exercise.

In a study published in the *Journal of Nutrition* fifty overweight women confirmed that a high-protein diet provided greater fat loss than a low-calorie, high-carbohydrate diet. When the high-protein diet is combined with exercise, there's an additive effect. More weight is lost, along with more fat instead of muscle.

In the study, all the women had a BMI of 33 kg/m2. Some women consumed a protein-rich diet containing specific levels of leucine, one of the essential amino acids for four months. The other women followed a diet based on the U.S. Food Guide Pyramid; their diet contained higher amounts of carbohydrates. Both groups consumed the same number of calories. The first group substituted protein foods, for example meat, dairy products, eggs, and nuts, for foods high in carbohydrates, such as breads, rice, cereal, pasta, and potatoes. Both diets worked, because when we restrict calories, we lose weight. But the women on the higher-protein diet lost more weight.

The subjects were required to follow one of two different exercise programs. The first plan involved walking two to three times a week. The second plan included five 30-minute walking sessions and two 30-minute weight-lifting sessions per week.

In both groups, the exercise helped spare lean muscle tissue and target fat loss. But the protein-rich, high-exercise group lost more weight, and almost 100 percent of the weight lost was fat.

The protein-rich diet is thought to work well because it contains a high level of leucine. The amino acid works with insulin to stimulate protein synthesis in muscle. The extra protein in this diet reduces muscle loss, while the low-carbohydrate component reduces insulin production, allowing the body to burn fat.

Whey protein also promotes the formation of glutathione, an antioxidant, which plays a key role in supporting the immune system.

Whey Good Supplements for Diabetics

The whey fraction of milk proteins has been identified as having significant health benefits, especially in weight management and insulin secretion effects. The exact mechanism is not known, but elevated levels of certain amino acids and hormones in whey, or formed during the digestion of whey protein, are possible explanations. It is known that proteins vary in to their effect on glucose metabolism. It has even been hypothesized that whey's effects on insulin might be similar to the effects of those pharmaceuticals that stimulate normal blood sugar levels in diabetics.

A new study published in the *American Journal of Clinical Nutrition* in 2005 showed that taking a whey supplement with meals can help stimulate insulin release in type 2 diabetics. The study tested the effects of adding whey to a meal of high-glycemic index breakfast or lunch. The insulin responses were 31 percent higher after breakfast (white bread) and 57 percent higher after lunch (mashed potatoes and meatballs) when whey was included in the meal than when it was not. The findings suggest that whey supplements could help diabetics improve their blood sugar control.

Another study, published in the *American Journal of Clinical Nutrition*, found that consuming a protein hydrolysate and amino acid mixture with carbohydrates increases insulin production in type 2 diabetics, and could therefore help control their blood sugar levels after a meal. Insulin responses were 299 percent higher in the diabetics and 132 percent higher in the control subjects after ingestion of the protein-enriched drink. The diabetics had an average 28 percent lower blood sugar response after consuming this drink than when they drank only the carbohydrate drink.

Whey Protein and Ingredient Labels
To make sure you are getting the important benefits of whey protein, always check the ingredient label before you buy a product. The first or second ingredient on the label should be:

• Whey protein isolate
• Whey protein concentrate

If the ingredient label says "protein blend, whey proteins may or may not be an ingredient. You have no way of knowing what the concentration level of the protein is. If the label says "hydrolyzed protein, the protein in this product may be a protein of lesser quality, such as gelatin protein. Check further to be sure the products have an acceptable amount of whey protein.

HOW MUCH IS TOO MUCH PROTEIN?

Although we have been discussing the importance of protein for weight loss and for promoting insulin sensitivity, I need to clarify the dangers of eating too much protein. As mentioned earlier, Leslie Beck recommends 0.5 to 0.8 g/pound of body weight if you are trying to lose weight and are physically active. This is by no means considered a high-protein diet (it's more a moderate-protein diet). I also encourage the consumption of significant dietary fiber with other low-glycemic carbohydrate choices and the combination of the right types of polyunsaturated fats.

High-protein, high-fat diets promote protein intakes of 28 to 65 percent of energy, and they severely limit carbohydrates. Such diets induce metabolic ketosis (using fat, instead of carbohydrates, for energy) and are popular because it induces quick weight loss. This initial weight loss may be attributed in part to the diuretic effect of a low-carbohydrate intake and its effects on sodium and water loss, glycogen (stored carbohydrate) depletion, and ketosis. As the diet is sustained, loss of appetite associated with ketosis leads to lower total caloric intake. High-protein diets that recommend more than thirty percent of calories from protein also can promote a negative energy balance due to significant restriction in the type and amount of foods eaten. The efficacy and the safety of these diets have not been documented in long-term studies.

The amount of protein recommended in high-protein diet regimens exceeds established requirements and may impose significant health risks. First, animal protein (rather than plant-based proteins, which also contain carbohydrates) is generally advocated in these diets. A diet rich in animal protein, saturated fat, and cholesterol raises LDL cholesterol levels, an effect that is compounded when high-carbohydrate, high-fiber plant foods that help cholesterol are limited. High-carbohydrate diets that include fruits, vegetables, nonfat dairy products, and whole grains have been shown to lower blood pressure, so limiting the consumption of these foods may also raise blood pressure. Extra protein in the system also increases urinary calcium loss, which may facilitate osteoporosis. In addition, elimination or severe restriction of fruit, vegetables, beans, and whole grains from the diet may increase cancer risk. A very high-protein diet is especially risky for people with diabetes because it can speed the progression, even for short lengths of time, of diabetic renal disease. Finally, because food choices may be severely restricted on high-protein diets, healthful foods such as low-fat milk products, cereals, grains, fruits, and vegetables (higher in carbohydrates and containing essential nutrients) are also generally restricted or eliminated. This can lead to deficiencies in essential vitamins, minerals, and fiber over the long term.

PROTEIN YOUR WAY

Overall total protein intake should not be excessive and should be reasonably proportional to the carbohydrates and fat consumed daily. The selected protein foods should be a mixture of high-quality animal proteins (egg, chicken, turkey), plant proteins, and whey protein supplements to limit total fat, saturated fat, and cholesterol.

WHAT YOU HAVE LEARNED IN THIS CHAPTER

- High-quality protein is essential for building muscles, losing weight, and improving insulin sensitivity.
- Protein requirements range from 0.36 grams per pound up to 0.8 grams per pound of body weight, depending on your activity level.
- Protein should be balanced in each meal and snack and should be consumed 5 to 6 times per day.
- Incorporate whey protein supplements into your day: one protein shake in the morning and one before dinner.

In the next chapter we will look at how obesity is one of the petals of the metabolic syndrome daisy and how carrying excess weight puts you at a greater risk for developing metabolic syndrome.

Chapter 6

_____

OBESITY AND OVERWEIGHT:
Our Growing Waistlines

In previous chapters we have looked at the growing conditions of metabolic syndrome, focusing primarily on dietary changes, from what our ancestors used to eat to the modern-day diet. Changes in fat, protein, and carbohydrate consumption have a significant impact on insulin resistance. These dietary changes have also led to the obesity epidemic that is now an urgent and growing problem in North America. Virtually all obese people are insulin resistant—and insulin resistance is the underlying cause of metabolic syndrome. Obesity, one of the components of metabolic syndrome, is one of the petals of the metabolic syndrome daisy.

A GROWING ISSUE

Obesity is the most common nutritional disorder in the industrialized world today. There are ominous statistics everywhere we turn:

- The rates of obesity are climbing, and the percentage of children and adolescents who are obese has doubled in the past twenty years.
- Some researchers have estimated that obesity causes about 300,000 deaths in the United States annually.
- Obesity is fueling an epidemic of type 2 diabetes, which reduces lifespan.

- The prevalence of obesity in U.S. adults has increased about fifty percent per decade since 1980.
- According to a *New England Journal of Medicine* report, studies suggest that two-thirds of American adults are overweight—they have a body mass index (BMI) of 25 or more—or obese—they have a BMI of 30 or more.
- Thirty percent of adults age twenty and older are obese.
- Fifteen percent of children age six to eleven and thirty percent age twelve to nineteen are obese.
- Obesity costs $117 billion a year.

ARE YOU OVERWEIGHT?

Obesity is a condition of excessive body fat that results from an energy imbalance, where intake of calories exceeds expenditure. Excess body fat increases the risk for premature death from heart disease, stroke, type 2 diabetes, and some cancers.

According to the World Health Organization (WHO), the best way to determine an overweight or obese adult is by using the body mass index (BMI), which uses weight in kilograms divided by the square of height in meters (Kglm²), or weight in pounds multiplied by 705, then divided twice by height in inches. A BMI between 25 and 29.9 indicates that an individual is overweight; an obese adult has a BMI of 30 or higher. The higher the BMI, the greater the risk of developing additional health problems. Overweight and obese individuals are at increased risk of developing metabolic syndrome, insulin resistance, heart disease, high blood pressure, stroke, diabetes, and many forms of cancer.

One variable the BMI fails to consider is lean body mass (tissue, bone, and muscle), which weighs significantly more than fat does. It is possible for a healthy, muscular individual to be classified as obese using the BMI formula. If you are a trained athlete, your weight based on a measured percentage of body fat would be a better indicator of what you should weigh. A normal healthy man should not exceed fifteen percent body fat, while the healthy limit for a woman is fifteen to twenty-two percent.

To calculate your BMI, check the table provided. Find your height in inches (remember there are twelve inches in a foot) along the left side. Move to the column with your weight in pounds. At the top of that column table is your BMI.

If your BMI is 24 or less, congratulations, you are within a healthy weight. However if you are above 25 then follow the graph back and find your ideal weight for height at a BMI of 24. (in other words, for a BMI of 24, my weight should be __.) This will give you a weight goal to work toward.

Table 6.1: Body Weight Classifications in Adults

Body Mass Index	Classification	Descriptor
<18.5	Underweight	May be associated with health problems for some people
18.5 to 24.9	Normal weight	Good weight for most people
25.0 to 29.9	Overweight	Increasing risk of developing health problems
>30	Obese	High risk of developing health problems

Source: World Health Organization, Obesity: Preventing and Managing the Global Epidemic, WHO technical report series no. 894 (Geneva: World Health Organization, 2000); Health Canada, Canadian Guidelines for Body Weight Classification in Adults (Ottawa: Health Canada 2003).

The BMI is an important tool for determining health risk. However, other factors, such as diet and lifestyle, can also affect health. If your BMI is in a healthy range, you should still be following the diet advice provided in this book to ensure you are achieving optimal health.

Table 6.2: BMI Calculations

BMI H (in)	19	20	21	22	23	24	25	26	27	28	29	30	31	32	33	34	35	36	37	38	39	40	41	42	43	44	45
													Weight (lbs)														
58	91	96	100	105	110	115	119	124	129	134	138	143	148	153	158	162	167	172	177	181	186	191	196	201	205	210	215
59	94	99	104	109	114	119	124	128	133	138	143	148	153	158	163	168	173	178	183	188	193	198	203	208	212	217	222
60	97	102	107	112	118	123	128	133	138	143	148	153	158	163	168	174	179	184	189	194	199	204	209	215	220	225	230
61	100	106	111	116	122	127	132	137	143	148	153	158	164	169	174	180	185	190	195	201	206	211	217	222	227	232	238
62	104	109	115	120	126	131	136	142	147	153	158	164	169	175	180	186	191	196	202	207	213	218	224	229	235	240	246
63	107	113	118	124	130	135	141	146	152	158	163	169	175	180	186	191	197	203	208	214	220	225	231	237	242	248	254
64	110	116	122	128	134	140	145	151	157	163	169	174	180	186	192	197	204	209	215	221	227	232	238	244	250	256	262
65	114	120	126	132	138	144	150	156	162	168	174	180	186	192	198	204	210	216	222	228	234	240	246	252	258	264	270
66	118	124	130	136	142	148	155	161	167	173	179	186	192	198	204	210	216	223	229	235	241	247	253	260	266	272	278
67	121	127	134	140	146	153	159	166	172	178	185	191	198	204	211	217	223	230	236	242	249	255	261	268	274	280	287
68	125	131	138	144	151	158	164	171	177	184	190	197	203	210	216	223	230	236	243	249	256	262	269	276	282	289	295
69	128	135	142	149	155	162	169	176	182	189	196	203	209	216	223	230	236	243	250	257	263	270	277	284	291	297	304
70	132	139	146	153	160	167	174	181	188	195	202	209	216	222	229	236	243	250	257	264	271	278	285	292	299	306	313
71	136	143	150	157	165	172	179	186	193	200	208	215	222	229	236	243	250	257	265	272	279	286	293	301	308	315	322
72	140	147	154	162	169	177	184	191	199	206	213	221	228	235	242	250	258	265	272	279	287	294	302	309	316	324	331
73	144	151	159	166	174	182	189	197	204	212	219	227	235	242	250	257	265	272	280	288	295	302	310	318	325	333	340
74	148	155	163	171	179	186	194	202	210	218	225	233	241	249	256	264	272	280	287	295	303	311	319	326	334	342	350
75	152	160	168	176	184	192	200	208	216	224	232	240	248	256	264	272	279	287	295	303	311	319	327	335	343	351	359
76	156	164	172	180	189	197	205	213	221	230	238	246	254	263	271	279	287	295	304	312	320	328	336	344	353	361	369

(Table adapted from the National Institutes of Health)

APPLE GONE BAD? TRY A PEAR!

Figure 6.1: Apple or Pear?

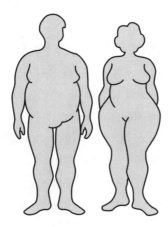

There is considerable variability in the relationship between obesity and chronic disease. Individuals with an "apple," or abdominal, fat distribution are at a substantially higher risk of developing cardiovascular and metabolic diseases than those with a "pear," or lower body, fat distribution pattern. Big hips are better than a big stomach, especially when it comes to heart disease, insulin resistance, and diabetes. Although genetics plays a major role in determining body shape, gender and age are also important factors. Men typically end up with the spare tire, or belly fat, and women usually gain excess weight around the buttocks. After menopause, as estrogen supplies dwindle, women start storing fat around their abdomens, becoming more apple-shaped and increasing their risk of cardiovascular disease and metabolic syndrome.

Waist-to-Hip Ratio

One way to determine if you're an apple or a pear is to find out your waist-to-hip ratio by dividing your waist measurement (at the narrowest point) by your hip measurement (at the widest point). Women with waist-to-hip ratios of more than 0.8 and men with waist-to-hip ratios of more than 1.0 are apples and are at an increased health risk because of their fat distribution.

All people who are obese are, to some degree, insulin resistant. However, people with abdominal obesity are far more insulin resistant. Why? One hypothesis is that the fat tissue from the abdominal region is more metabolically relevant.

WHITE FAT, BROWN FAT, NO FAT

Thermogenesis is the creation of heat in the body. The food we eat provides us with energy that is measured in calories. When the body burns calories (regardless of whether we are sleeping or running), heat is produced.

White fat is the insulating layer of fat just beneath the skin that buffers you from the cold and stores calories. Brown fat is the metabolically active fat that surrounds your organs and cushions the blood vessels and spinal column. You can't see brown fat, but it is the fat your body burns to create heat; brown fat does not store calories. The heat, in addition to keeping you warm, burns white fat for energy. You may have noticed after eating a large meal, you start to sweat. This is called diet-induced thermogenesis. A portion of the food you eat is converted into heat, and the rest is metabolized, absorbed, and stored.

Brown fat, the fat in the abdominal region, is more metabolically relevant because it creates obstacles for insulin action. There is a stronger link between intra-abdominal fat and insulin resistance than between overall obesity and insulin resistance. Men have higher levels of intra-abdominal fat than women do—in fact, women have one half the level. Even though women have more total body fat than men because their fat is primarily subcutaneous, they don't have the rates of metabolic syndrome and heart disease men have. Abdominal obesity and insulin resistance have a dual relationship. Abdominal obesity stimulates insulin resistance, and insulin resistance promotes weight gain.

Thermogenesis and brown fat activity explain why one person can eat all day without gaining an ounce while another person can gain weight just thinking about food. Thin people have activated brown fat, while overweight or apple-shaped individuals have dormant brown fat. It is essential to make dietary changes that will stimulate the activity of brown fat to prevent insulin resistance by allowing insulin to do its job properly. The best thing a person can do is avoid becoming obese in the first place. Losing weight and preventing further weight gain will help people who are already overweight or obese.

CAUSES OF OBESITY

The causes of obesity are not fully understood. However, it is known that there are several factors, some very simple and others very complicated. The most important causes are:

• Genetics
• Sedentary lifestyle
• Sleep
• Stress
• High-caloric diet
• Sympathetic nervous system
• Hormone imbalance

Genetics

There are complex interactions between genes and our environment. Obesity would not be possible if the human genome did not have the genes for it. Genes make obesity possible, but eating too many calories over time will increase the potential for obesity. Genetic contributions are estimated to contribute from 20 to 75 percent of variability in body weight and composition within the population. Gene mutations, such as leptin, leptin receptor, and PPAR gamma, have been identified as causes of obesity. One study published in the *New England Journal of Medicine* found that of 121 obese subjects, 4 had a mutation in the gene PPAR gamma. None of the 237 subjects of normal weight had the mutation, confirming that gene mutations may be a potential cause of obesity.

The "thrifty gene hypothesis" suggests that people developed strong biological mechanisms for conserving energy as fat to enable their survival in times of famine. In times of plenty, such as the present day in the developed world, the thrifty genes promote obesity. The complex gene-environment interaction is clearly implicated in the obesity epidemic, as the rapid increase in obesity suggests an environment that promotes obesity. According to the WHO, however, the fundamental cause of the obesity epidemic is societal: our environment promotes inactive lifestyles, and we consume too many calories.

Sedentary Lifestyle

People are eating too much for their activity level. Sedentary lifestyle is one of the principal causes of obesity. And it has been proven that physical activity is one of the best ways to utilize the body's energy.

An increase in physical activity allows the intake of more calories and achieves a more favorable caloric balance in the body; activity is a good way to avoid obesity. Data from the Third National Health and Nutrition Examination Survey reports no physical activity in 25 percent of the population, and no regular activity at all in an additional 44 percent. To add to the problem, participation in daily, school-based physical education is declining. Current recommendations for health benefit are more than sixty minutes of physical activity per day. Physical activity among children is negatively associated with overweight and obesity, while TV viewing and video game use increase risk of excess weight. In 2002, average hours of television viewing per week for all Canadians older than twelve was 21.8; Americans older than twelve watched an average of 28 hours per week.

The Nurse's Health Study conducted in the United States from 1992 to 1998 documented new cases of obesity and diabetes among subjects and correlated outcomes with sedentary behaviors. Each two-hour per day increment in television watching was associated with a 23 percent increase in obesity and a 14 percent increase in the risk of diabetes. The authors of the study also noted that each one-hour per day of brisk walking was associated with a 24 percent reduction in obesity and a 34 percent reduction in the risk of diabetes. The study findings support the premise that decreasing sedentary behaviors and increasing active leisure time reduces the risk of obesity.

We will discuss physical activity in greater detail in Chapter 11.

Sleep

Sleep deprivation is increasingly being linked to the obesity epidemic. Research shows that obese people sleep less than their normal-weight peers. Insufficient sleep has been associated with changes in hormone levels that may stimulate appetite. In a study published in *Archives of Internal Medicine* in 2005, people with a normal BMI slept sixteen minutes more per day than obese people. Even an extra twenty minutes of shut-eye can be beneficial. Those who slept less were also found to have fifteen per cent less leptin, a hormone that suppresses appetite.

Stress

The relationship between stress and obesity is a much-studied problem. Our stressful lifestyles may be influencing the rise in obesity. The hormone cortisol is secreted by the adrenal glands in response to physical, psychological, or environmental stress. When we experience chronic stress, our cortisol levels will remain elevated. Research now correlates chronically elevated cortisol levels with blood sugar problems, fat accumulation, fat cells' resistance to fat loss, fatigue, and heart disease. Certain cases of obesity have clear clinical features of high cortisol levels, including a middle-fat distribution of excess body-fat mass, elevated blood pressure, insulin resistance, and high cholesterol and triglycerides.

When we have high cortisol levels, we often require adrenal support. Many people are suffering from exhausted adrenal glands.

High-Caloric Diet

Eating more calories than we burn in a day causes the caloric balance to accumulate. Although that is fairly easy to understand, what is more difficult is why obesity is such a huge problem considering the public's growing awareness of it and its associated health problems.

Data from the United States and Canada show that food consumption is increasing, and there have been overall increases in soft-drink consumption and sugar consumption. In surveys of children in grades 6 and 7, sweetened soft-drink consumption was associated with increased BMI and frequency obesity. Data suggest that fat consumption is decreasing.

The increase in eating food away from home, particularly in fast-food restaurants, is not surprising, considering that in the United States, the number of fast-food restaurants grew 147% from 1972 to 1995, and the percentage of meals and snacks consumed at fast-food restaurants doubled. Eating at fast-food restaurants is associated with increased calorie and fat intake largely due to increases in high-fat, high-sugar food choices such as French fries and soft drinks, and decreases in consumption of fruits, vegetables, and milk. Even our grocery store environments have changed. The change from small grocery stores in neighborhoods to large supermarkets has been positively associated with increased caloric intake because the supermarkets offer a greater variety of processed and convenience foods.

An increase in calories consumed can also be partly blamed on larger portion sizes. Examinations of trends in food portion sizes in the United States from 1977 to 1998 revealed that portion sizes and energy intake increased for all key foods (except pizza) at all locations, with the largest portions consumed at fast-food restaurants. "Super sizing" of portions is one of the greatest contributors. For example, the current McDonald's "child-size" soft drink is twelve ounces; the same serving size in the 1950s would have been marketed as "king-size." A study comparing the USDA's recommended serving size and what is currently being sold in the marketplace revealed that serving sizes now exceed the standards: soda by 35%; fast-food hamburgers by 112%; bagels by 195%; steak by 224%; and cookies by 700%. Portion sizes began to grow in the 1970s, although fewer than ten large-sized portions were introduced in that decade. The number of larger sizes rose sharply in the 1980s and has continued to increase steadily. Between 1995 and 1999, sixty-five new large-size portions were introduced.

Exposure to food advertising may also influence the purchase of foods with more calories and less nutritional value. Foods that are heavily advertised are generally overconsumed relative to recommendations, while foods that are advertised less frequently are underconsumed. We don't see many television commercials for fruits and vegetables, but there are numerous ones for fast-food restaurants and soft drinks. In 1997 (the most recent report), U.S. food manufacturers and retailers spent $11 billion in mass-marketing media advertising. This amount included $765 million on confectionaries and snacks, $571 million on McDonald's, $549 million on soft drinks, and $105 million on fruits and vegetables. The entire nutrition education budget for the USDA that same year was $333 million (or three percent of food industry expenditures). These food advertisements generally reflect the types of foods being consumed; these foods represent an increased risk of obesity, dental cavities, cardiovascular disease, and type 2 diabetes.

Marketing of food is not limited to advertising. An interesting case is soft-drink marketing in schools. Competition among soft-drink companies led to "pouring rights" contracts with universities and school districts in the 1990s. These contracts involve large lump-sum payments to schools in return for exclusive rights to sell the company's products in vending machines and at all school events. On the surface, this arrangement appears mutually beneficial. Schools benefit from funds that enable the purchase of supplies, such as computers, which might not be possible otherwise, and soft-drink companies instill brand loyalty among children while increasing market share and profit. Such arrangements, however, place schools in the unusual position of "pushing" soft-drink consumption, which encourages unhealthy dietary practices. Now, many schools across the United States and Canada are trying to reverse these contracts, and there is a push toward getting rid of all vending and soft drink machines in schools. Conveniences such as vending machines have been blamed for the increasing obesity trend.

Sympathetic Nervous System

The sympathetic nervous system is the part of the nervous system that speeds the heart and initiates other physiological reactions to prepare the body to deal with stress. It plays a critical role in metabolism and cardiovascular health.

Researchers have found that some obese people have increased sympa-thetic nervous system activity; it is increased in those people with high levels of brown fat, or intra-abdominal fat. The apple body-fat distribution pattern shows excessive fat around the abdomen, whereas the pear shape exhibits subcutaneous white fat in the buttocks and thighs. This may explain why apple-shaped people have an increased risk of virtually all diseases, especially metabolic syndrome.

Hormone Imbalance

Hormones have a powerful influence on weight gain and obesity. Products of adipocytes (fat cells) play a role in the insulin resistance associated with obesity and metabolic syndrome. Fat cells secrete leptin, a hormone that is thought to cause satiety, the feeling of having eaten enough, and stimulates the metabolic rate. Another hormone, ghrelin, is a powerful appetite-stimulating hormone and has been found in very high concentrations in the central nervous system of obese individuals. Adiponectin is important because it stimulates insulin sen-sitivity and has anti-inflammatory effects, two of the central effects required in the prevention of metabolic syndrome. Obese people and those with metabolic syndrome secrete less adiponectin than do people who are not obese. Working in just the opposite fashion is resistan, which decreases insulin sensitivity. The ideal scenario is to have high levels of adiponectin and leptin, and low levels of ghrelin and resistan.

Free fatty acids are the primary breakdown of fat cell nutrient stores. Obesity increases levels of free fatty acids. The overall release of free fatty acids into the bloodstream is also a function of fat mass. An obese person will have higher total free fatty acid release than a thin person, even if each fat cell is releasing the same quantity of free fatty acids. This may contribute to higher circulating free fatty acid levels and insulin resistance in obese people. The adverse effects of high levels of free fatty acids extend beyond insulin resistance. Circulating free fatty acids can be used as fuel, or they can be con-verted into triglycerides, which can lead to high blood triglyceride levels, one of the risk factors for cardiovascular disease.

THE ROLE OF OBESITY IN METABOLIC SYNDROME

Figure 6.2: Metabolic Syndrome: The Role of Obesity

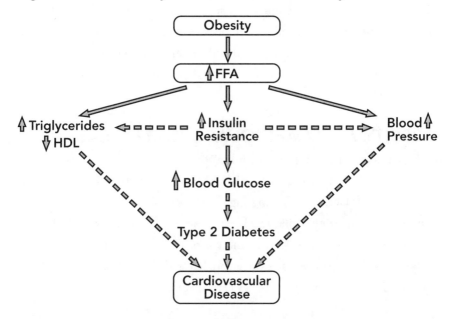

Obesity, especially abdominal obesity, plays a large role in the development of metabolic syndrome. Obesity is a multifactorial disease involving interactions among genetic, hormonal, metabolic, environmental, and cultural factors. Metabolism is often slowed down in obesity. The energy intake outbalances the energy expenditure, and excess energy is accumulated as fat. The body has limited capacity to store carbohydrates, but virtually unlimited fat storage capacity.

As mentioned above, obese people have increased levels of free fatty acids, which in turn increase insulin resistance. Insulin resistance is correlated with obesity and can be reversed with weight loss. High circulating insulin levels (because our cells aren't able to properly utilize the insulin) lead to increased blood pressure, increased triglycerides, decreased HDL (good cholesterol), and increased blood glucose levels, which in turn lead to type 2 diabetes. High blood pressure, elevated triglycerides, decreased HDL, and type 2 diabetes are all directly linked to cardiovascular disease. Collectively these risk factors are now known as metabolic syndrome.

All components of the metabolic syndrome can be modified through lifestyle changes. A recent clinical trial found that weight loss reduced the incidence of the metabolic syndrome in obese individuals. Weight loss of 6.5% was achieved over a four-week period with the use of a very low-calorie diet. After four weeks, the prevalence of the metabolic syndrome was reduced, and improvements of all the individual components were achieved.

OBESITY AND CARDIOVASCULAR DISEASE

Obesity is a major risk factor for cardiovascular disease (CVD). The overall risk of CVD increases with increasing BMI, and a high BMI is associated with CVD risk factors, including high blood pressure, high total and LDL cholesterol, high triglyceride levels, and low HDL cholesterol. Both BMI and waist-hip ratio have been predictive of CVD risk factors, although a higher waist-hip ratio was a stronger predictor than BMI. Losing weight is associated with improvements in CVD risk factors.

OBESITY AND TYPE 2 DIABETES

Of all common diseases, type 2 diabetes appears to be most directly correlated with increasing obesity. BMI is a powerful predictor of diabetes risk. Globally, the increasing prevalence of type 2 diabetes closely follows the increasing prevalence of obesity.

Once termed "adult-onset diabetes," type 2 diabetes is being diagnosed in younger people as childhood obesity increases. Lifestyle changes, including dietary changes and increased activity levels, will help prevent type 2 diabetes.

WHAT YOU HAVE LEARNED IN THIS CHAPTER

- Obesity is a growing epidemic affecting 63% of people in the United States and is fueling the progression of type 2 diabetes.

- A BMI greater than 25 is classified as overweight; a BMI of more than 30 is obese.
- There are numerous causes of obesity, including genetics, sedentary life-style, sleep, stress, hormone imbalance, high-calorie diet, and sympathetic nervous system abnormalities.
- Weight loss is one of the key components to improving metabolic syndrome parameters, cardiovascular disease risk factors, and type 2 diabetes.

In the next chapter we will learn more about insulin resistance, and how to prevent it from becoming type 2 diabetes.

PART III

THE ROOT
TO THE LEAF

Chapter 7

INSULIN RESISTANCE LEADS TO TYPE 2 DIABETES

In Part II we looked at diet and how choosing the wrong types of food can lead to insulin resistance. Insulin resistance is one of the most serious metabolic abnormalities linked to numerous chronic diseases. The root of metabolic syndrome is insulin resistance, a condition in which the body does not efficiently use insulin, so the pancreas has to make a lot more insulin to regulate blood glucose, the simple sugar that is the main source of energy for the body's cells.

But your cells cannot use glucose without insulin. After you consume carbohydrates, your blood sugar levels rise. As the regulator of blood sugar levels, insulin's job is to push the glucose into the cells. On the surface of the cells are insulin receptors, which act like little doors that open and close to regulate the inflow of blood sugar. When the body is continually blasted by foods containing high levels of simple sugars, the cells are bombarded with so much insulin that these doors begin to malfunction and shut down. With fewer doors open, the body needs to produce even more insulin to push glucose into the cells. Insulin left free in the bloodstream cannot perform its function of lowering sugar levels. The pancreas is stimulated by sugar's continued presence to produce more insulin, and a vicious cycle is in place, resulting in a condition called insulin resistance.

With insulin resistance, the blood insulin levels are chronically high, which inhibits our fat cells from giving up their energy stores to let us lose weight. The more overweight we are, the more resistant to insulin we tend to become. This happens because extra fat causes a hormone reaction that closes the cells' doors to incoming glucose. High insulin leads to more fat cells (inefficient burners of glucose) and fewer lean muscle cells; more fat cells mean more weight, less ability or desire to exercise, and therefore less glucose burned. This is why some people gain more weight than others. However, the good news is that as we lose body fat, the insulin resistance improves.

To understand why insulin is such a critical component to the metabolic syndrome, it is important to understand the relationship between food, blood sugar, insulin, and fat.

INSULIN TRIGGERS FAT STORAGE

Glucagon, another hormone secreted by the pancreas, works in much the same manner as insulin, except in the opposite direction. If blood glucose is high, then no glucagon is secreted. When blood glucose becomes low, however (for example between meals and during exercise), more and more glucagon is secreted. Like insulin, glucagon has an effect on many cells of the body, most notably the liver. The effect of glucagon is to make the liver release the glucose it has stored in its cells into the bloodstream, with the net effect of increasing blood glucose.

If we have more glucose in our bodies than our cells need, insulin takes extra blood glucose and transports it into fat storage. Our bodies have a limited capacity to store carbohydrates—that is why it is so important to eat only those carbohydrates that can be burned by our bodies. Once the extra sugar is transported into fat storage, blood sugar levels return to normal. When blood sugar levels don't return to normal, this is diabetes.

Figure 7.1: Normal Glucose and Insulin Response

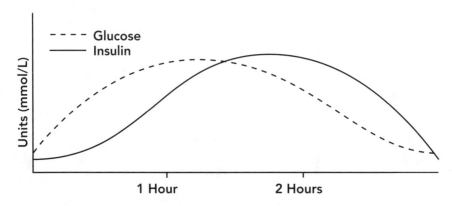

Figure 7.1 shows the normal rises and falls of blood sugar and insulin levels after eating carbohydrates. The insulin rises in the middle to normalize blood sugar levels. It is during this spike that the body makes and stores fat. The body can actually make fat as quickly as two to three hours after eating a high-carbohydrate food. Keeping insulin levels from spiking is the key to weight loss and preventing metabolic syndrome. In Chapter 10 you will learn how to balance your insulin levels by consuming protein with your carbohydrates and by choosing the appropriate types of carbohydrates.

HYPOGLYCEMIA

Glucose is the exclusive fuel of the human nervous system and the primary fuel of most systems in the body. A healthy level of glucose in the blood is therefore essential to life and health. Hypoglycemia means low blood sugar. This usually occurs when the pancreas oversecretes insulin, resulting in a rapid absorption of sugar.

Hypoglycemia can cause shakiness, dizziness, tiredness, mental dullness, headaches, intense cravings for sugary or starchy foods, irritability, depression, night sweats, and nervous habits. Most of us suffer from hypoglycemia to a certain extent—think about the way you feel around three in the afternoon when you are tired, hungry, and craving sugar, needing that chocolate fix. These are all very common reactions of hypoglycemia. Elevated stress levels may also contribute to this condition. Though hypoglycemia can be inherited, dietary factors are usually the main contributor. Although it may seem paradoxical, low blood sugar can also be an early sign of diabetes. The prolonged stress of compensating for the blood sugar swings contributes to the development of diabetes.

FROM HIGH TO LOW

When excess sugar goes into the bloodstream (which is the case in most North Americans' diets because of an overconsumption of sugar and carbohydrates), the pancreas reacts instantly by releasing a large quantity of insulin into the blood. Since this is an "emergency" release, the insulin is generally in excess of what is required to maintain a steady level, and too much sugar is removed from the blood. When the blood sugar level drops below the threshold level, a different panic response is triggered because a low blood sugar level is a serious crisis in the body. This response causes the adrenal glands to release glucocorticoid hormones, which convert glycogen in the liver and muscle tissues into glucose. This causes the glucose level to rise again and, since this was a panic response, the glucose level will likely exceed its base level, triggering yet another insulin release. The swing from high to low may continue for many hours.

This is exactly what is observed in someone during a glucose tolerance test. In a glucose tolerance test, people fast for eight to twelve hours, have a blood sample taken to determine their baseline, then swallow 75 grams of glucose. The blood sugar level is taken at half-hour to one-hour intervals for the next several hours. In an individual demonstrating the reactive hypoglycemia response, the glucose levels will rise sharply within a half hour. The rise is followed by a sharp drop, and in the one- to two-hour interval the blood sugar will be sharply lower. At this point serious mood changes such as irritability are demonstrated; when the blood sugar levels rise, the mood and behavior return to normal. The same response occurs when large amounts of refined sugar are consumed, although the response is not as extreme. The pattern of blood sugar swings contributes to the development of obesity and cumulative stress on the pancreas, adrenal glands, and liver.

These symptoms are not normal. The best way to deal with them is to eat regularly throughout the day so your body does not have surges in blood sugar and insulin. Regular eating will prevent you from getting too hungry, will keep your blood sugar from dropping too low, and will help you lose weight.

Figure 7.2 shows the glucose and insulin response of someone with insulin resistance that has resulted in hypoglycemia. The insulin needs to spike to bring down the glucose levels. The glucose levels fall rapidly, causing hypoglycemia. People have varying degrees of hypoglycemia—in fact, severe hypoglycemia can be life-threatening. People with insulin resistance tend to store most carbohydrates as fat rather than use them as energy.

Figure 7.2: Hypoglycemic Response

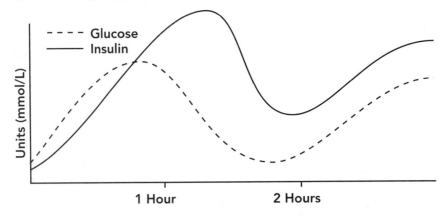

INSULIN RESISTANCE

In Chapter 2 we discussed the diet of our ancestors, who ate nuts, seeds, berries, green leafy vegetables, meat for protein, and virtually no grains or other carbohydrates. They ate few refined foods because refined foods weren't available. Now we are bombarded with processed and convenience foods, white sugar, white pasta, white, white, white everything! Our bodies are not designed to handle the abundance of these types of carbohydrates. After our bodies reach their capacity to use carbohydrates, they convert them into fat storage mode, which, coupled with our sedentary lifestyle, is a recipe for overweight and obesity. This refined carbohydrate overload leads to the development of insulin resistance.

Figure 7.3 shows the insulin and glucose response in a person with insulin resistance. It is a vicious cycle in which glucose from carbohydrates invades the bloodstream, insulin is then released and rises, which causes hypoglycemia. Hypoglycemia makes you crave more carbohydrates. More carbohydrates make glucose, glucose needs insulin, and the cycle never ends.

Figure 7.3: Insulin and Glucose Response in Someone with Insulin Resistance

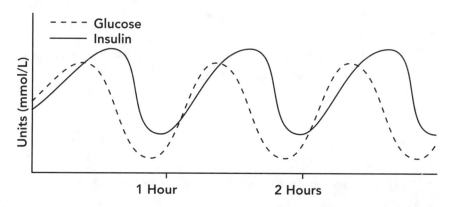

Ideally, insulin should gently roll up and down all day long in low hills without any dramatic high spikes—that type of insulin response will help promote fat loss. (See Figure 7.1.)

Do You Have Insulin Resistance?

The diagnosis of insulin resistance is fairly simple. Place a check by any items that apply to you.

Do you have or are you:

• A family history of diabetes, overweight, abnormal cholesterol or triglycerides, high blood pressure, or heart disease?
• Frequent cravings for sugary or starch foods?

- A difficult time losing weight, especially around your middle?
- The feeling that you are addicted to carbohydrates?
- Shakiness, difficulty thinking, or headaches (often in the afternoon) that go away after you eat?
- Afternoon fatigue?
- Hypoglycemia?
- A Body Mass Index (BMI) greater than 30? (See Chapter 9.)
- High blood pressure?
- High triglycerides and low HDL cholesterol?
- Forty-five years old or older?
- A history of gestational diabetes in pregnancy?
- Polycystic ovary syndrome?
- The skin changes called acanthosis—velvety, mossy, flat, warty-like, darkened skin on your neck or armpits or underneath the breasts?

Are you:
- Ten pounds or more over what you would call your "ideal weight"?
- Exercising less than two times per week?
- Of Native American, Asian, African-American, or Hispanic ancestry?
- A smoker?

If you answer yes to three or more of these questions, you are likely insulin resistant. The more yes answers, the more likely you are to have it. Did you check any of the items in the list below from Chapter 1? If you did, you likely have metabolic syndrome and are at an even greater risk of developing health problems such as type 2 diabetes and cardiovascular disease.

- High blood pressure
- Low HDL
- High LDL
- High triglycerides
- BMI greater than 30

- Abnormal glucose tolerance test
- Hypoglycemia symptoms

Diagnosing Insulin Resistance

If you have three or more of the health risks in the insulin resistance quiz, you should see your doctor and ask for a fasting insulin level test or a fasting blood glucose test to measure your blood glucose after you've been fasting for several hours. A fasting insulin level of more than 15 mmol/L is a flag for insulin resistance. A two-hour blood glucose test is the most accurate measure. For this test you drink 75 grams of glucose. Your blood is then drawn every few hours to monitor your insulin and blood glucose levels. People with insulin resistance have normal to low glucose levels and higher than normal insulin levels.

Our bodies want a blood glucose level between 4 mmol/L (70 mg/dL) and 7 mmol/L (110 mg/dl). Below 4 mmol/L (70 mg/dL) is considered hypo-glycemia. Above 7 mmol/L (110 mg/dL) can be normal if you have eaten in the past two or three hours. That is why the test measures your blood glucose while you are fasting. Your blood glucose should be between 4 mmol/L (70 mg/dL) and 7 mmol/L (110 mg/dL). If it is above 7 mmol/L (110mg/dL) then you are said to have impaired glucose tolerance, a risk factor for metabolic syndrome and diabetes. Even after you have eaten, however, your glucose should be below 7 mmol/L (110 mg/dL). Above 7 mmol/L (110 mg/dL) is considered hyperglycemia (too much glucose in the blood). If you have two blood sugar measurements above 11.1 mmol/L (200 mg/dL) after you have a sugar-water drink, then you have type 2 diabetes.

Controlling Insulin Resistance

There is no outright cure for insulin resistance. Fortunately, it's possible to control your insulin resistance. Such control will help with weight loss and can prevent other health problems. Dietary changes, exercise, and weight loss are the most important factors in dealing with insulin resistance. See Chapter 10 for a suggested food and energy plan. Natural supplements, which help control insulin levels, are discussed in Chapter 12.

What can be done to control insulin resistance?

- Limit your intake of simple carbohydrates and choose low-glycemic carbohydrates (see Chapter 4).
- Combine carbohydrates with a protein at every meal and snack.
- Eat five to six small meals per day.
- Replace one or two meals per day with a protein shake.
- Exercise regularly and include cardiovascular exercise and weight training. Controlling body fat is more important than losing pounds. Remember that muscle is more metabolically active than fat; even though you may be sitting doing nothing, muscle burns more calories than fat, so any increase in lean muscle will make your body a more efficient fat-burning machine.
- Use nutritional supplements (see Chapter 12.)

These actions are not optional or negotiable. Your body will burn fat (and properly utilize nutrients) only if its metabolism is balanced. These changes in your dietary and lifestyle regime are the only way to address the root problem—insulin resistance.

INSULIN AND CHRONIC DISEASE

Your metabolism is the food-processing and energy-production system of your body. It is made up of extremely fine-tuned internal processes. Insulin is the master hormone of your metabolism. When your metabolism is out of balance and your insulin levels are consistently elevated, a long list of deadly complications can result:

- Heart disease
- Hardening of the arteries
- Damage to artery walls
- Increased cholesterol levels
- Increased blood pressure
- Osteoporosis

- Vitamin and mineral deficiencies
- Kidney disease
- Fat-burning mechanism turned off
- Accumulation and storage of fat
- Weight gain

These disorders are all merely symptoms of a single basic disturbance in metabolism—excess insulin and insulin resistance.

Health experts now believe they have identified insulin resistance as the common factor explaining the increase in chronic diseases. A large study in 2004 of more than 39,000 people in forty countries made a connection between high blood sugar and cardiovascular disease. About half the subjects were men, averaging 63 years of age, and the researchers determined that only one man in three had normal glucose and insulin levels. One in five had diabetes that had gone undetected, and more than one in four had prediabetic readings. The study findings emphasize the importance of controlling blood sugar and regulating insulin levels.

Insulin resistance accounts for the otherwise higher number of overweight people in this country. The problem at its most basic is that the sugar not removed from the blood has to go somewhere. It is either stored as fat or converted to triglycerides. And as we all know, obesity and high triglycerides have many undesirable health effects. Out-of-control blood sugar is also a definition of diabetes.

INSULIN RESISTANCE AND CARDIOVASCULAR DISEASE

Insulin resistance results in abnormalities of blood lipids (cholesterol and triglycerides—high levels of triglycerides (>150 mg/dl) and low levels of HDL cholesterol (<40 mg/dl in men and <50 mg/dl in women). The relationship between insulin resistance and blood lipids has to do with the role insulin plays on the metabolism of free fatty acids. In insulin resistance, there is an increase in free fatty acids released from the adipocytes (fat cells). This increase causes the levels of free fatty acids to rise, which stimulates the synthesis of triglyceride production. This increase in triglycerides increases the cardiovascular disease risk in insulin-resistant individuals.

INSULIN RESISTANCE AND TYPE 2 DIABETES

Insulin resistance is present in virtually all cases of type 2 diabetes, yet it exists in many more individuals who do not yet have hyperglycemia but have metabolic syndrome (and are at risk for developing type 2 diabetes). Before they develop diabetes, people are able to hypersecrete insulin to maintain normal blood glucose levels. At some point, in people who develop type 2 diabetes, cells in the pancreas fail, insulin levels fall, and blood glucose levels rise. Unfortunately, it is only at this point (when fasting blood glucose levels increase) that prediabetes is diagnosed. Insulin resistance is often the last part of the metabolic syndrome to be diagnosed, even though it may be the underlying abnormality in people with the condition.

INSULIN RESISTANCE AND INFLAMMATION

Inflammation is the "buzz word" of the year and for good reason. However, inflammation is probably one of the least talked about risk factors for metabolic syndrome. The inflammation related to metabolic syndrome is chronic, it is invisible, and it exists throughout our bodies. Inflammation is the smoking gun that links excess body fat to today's epidemic rise in insulin resistance and metabolic syndrome.

Treatment and control of inflammation may reduce the risk of insulin resistance and thereby prevent metabolic syndrome and other related diseases. Although the relationship is complex, diet and nutrition, especially in the area of carbohydrate and fatty acid metabolism, have a significant impact on our bodies' inflammatory state.

Clinical data has suggested that inflammatory factors may be associated with insulin resistance. Several studies report elevated levels of C-reactive protein, white blood cell count, uric acid, and fibrinogen in people with insulin resistance or metabolic syndrome. The Third National Health and

Nutrition Examination Survey (NHANES III) examined the relationship between inflammatory markers and insulin resistance in nondiabetic U.S. adults. A strong positive relationship existed between inflammatory markers and insulin resistance. Many of these inflammatory markers, such as C-reactive protein and fibrinogen, also play an important role in the development of cardiovascular disease. Treatment of inflammation may reduce the risk of insulin resistance, diabetes, and related cardiovascular disease.

TYPE 2 DIABETES: THE EPIDEMIC

Excess body fat is one of the contributing factors to type 2 diabetes, and the rise in obesity has led to a higher incidence of this disease. In Canada, diabetes affects 1.5 million people, and another 750,000 have it and don't even know it. Diabetes affects more than 16 million Americans, approximately one-third of whom are undiagnosed. This number is also on the rise. From 1990 to 1998, the frequency of diabetes, especially type 2 diabetes in adults, increased by about 33%. Diabetes has been predicted to affect from 125 million to 333 million people worldwide by the year 2025. It is likely that the number of people with insulin resistance will be much greater than this estimate. The biggest percentage increases are projected to be among those aged 75 years and older. These predictions are consistent with the trend seen in virtually every developed nation, where diabetes ranks as one of the top two causes of blindness, renal failure, and lower limb amputation. Through its effects on the cardiovascular system (nearly 80% of diabetics with uncontrolled blood sugar levels—greater than 70 mg/dL or 4 mmol/L—die of cardiovascular disease), it is also now one of the leading causes of death.

There are two major types of diabetes: type 1 diabetes, or insulin-dependent diabetes, and type 2 diabetes, or non-insulin dependent diabetes. The primary defect in type 1 diabetes resides in the pancreas, resulting in insulin deficiency and the resulting failure to metabolize glucose. About 90% of diabetics have type 2 diabetes, in which insulin is generally present, but the cells' ability to respond to insulin and absorb glucose from the blood is impaired. This situation comes about because of the wear and tear on and abuse of the insulin/sugar-regulating process.

Most people with type 2 diabetes are overweight or obese. In fact, excess weight often precedes type 2 diabetes and is now a major risk factor for the development of type 2 diabetes. Symptoms of type 2 diabetes include insatiable appetite and thirst, frequent urination, light-headedness, blurred vision, numbness or tingling in the hands and toes, deep fatigue, irritability, and depression.

One of the best ways to prevent type 2 diabetes is to control insulin sensitivity/resistance. Another strategy is to remove or reduce the sugar/insulin stress.

Type 2 diabetes is really a severe case of insulin resistance, so the solution to the condition is to find a way to increase the sensitivity of cells to insulin and help the body get the sugar out of the blood and into the cells so it can be metabolized and turned into energy. (The inability to metabolize blood sugar is one of the reasons most diabetics often feel tired and fatigued.) We can improve insulin sensitivity by making dietary changes, including choosing low-glycemic carbohydrates and sufficient lean, high-quality protein; increasing consumption of omega-3s and monounsaturated fats, and reducing consumption of trans and saturated fats. Increasing physical activity levels is also a key element.

RISK FACTORS FOR DIABETES

The number-one most important risk factor for diabetes is excess body fat, especially around the middle. Overweight and obesity are the leading causes of type 2 diabetes. Even being just a few pounds overweight carries a significant increased risk for type 2 diabetes, and the greater the fat accumulation, the greater the likelihood of developing type 2 diabetes. Several population studies have demonstrated the link between the increased risk for type 2 diabetes and a high body mass index (BMI; see Chapter 6). In a report from the Nurse's Health Study, women with a BMI in the average range of 24 to 24.9 had an elevated risk, up to five times more than women with a BMI of 22. The risk of diabetes in patients with a BMI of 31 was forty times greater. The study also reported that changes in body weight could be a strong predictor of risk for diabetes. When compared with women of stable weight, women who gained 20 kg (44 lbs) or more during adulthood had a twelve times greater risk than the control group. In contrast, women who lost more than 20 kg (44 lbs) lowered their risk by nine times.

If you will recall our discussion on obesity in Chapter 6, hormones from fat cells play a significant role in the development of insulin resistance. Fat, not just body weight, carries the greatest risk for the development of diabetes. This is why even normal-weight people can develop type 2 diabetes if they have an increased body fat percentage, especially if that excess fat is around the middle. Fat cells secrete hormone compounds such as resistan, leptin, and free fatty acids, all of which dampen the effects of insulin.

As fat cells increase in number and size they cause a decrease in compounds that promote the action of insulin, thus leading to type 2 diabetes. Adiponectin is an important hormone that stimulates insulin sensitivity and has anti-inflammatory effects, two of the central effects required in the prevention of metabolic syndrome. Obese people and people with metabolic syndrome secrete less adiponectin than do people who are not obese.

Risk factors for type 2 diabetes:
- Family history of diabetes
- Obesity (BMI> 30)
- Increased waist/hip ratio
- Age (older than 45)
- Race/ethnicity (especially African-American, Hispanic American, Native American/Canadian, Asian American)
- Previously identified impaired fasting glucose or impaired glucose tolerance test
- High blood pressure
- High triglycerides
- Low adiponectin levels
- Elevated fasting insulin levels
- Polycystic ovary syndrome
- Inactive lifestyle—exercise less than twice per week
- Poor diet high in refined sugars, saturated fat
- Gestational diabetes (diabetes during pregnancy)

You will notice that the risk factors for type 2 diabetes are very similar to those of insulin resistance. That is because insulin resistance is essentially type 2 diabetes. However, you can correct insulin resistance (prediabetes) before it becomes full-blown diabetes. As we learned in Chapter 1, prediabetes is a warning light that danger is ahead and something must be done. That something involves dietary and lifestyle changes that will help reverse insulin resistance. See Chapter 1, Figure 1.2 for a reminder of the progression of type 2 diabetes.

Findings from the government's Third National Health and Nutrition Examination Survey (NHANES III) make it quite clear that diabetes is a disease of diet and lifestyle. According to the survey, 69 percent of those with type 2 diabetes did not exercise at all or didn't engage in any regular exercise activity; 62 percent ate fewer than five servings of fruits and vegetables per day; 65 percent consumed more than 30 percent of their daily calories from fat and more than 10 percent from saturated fat; and 82 percent were either overweight or obese.

The famous Physician's Health Study, which followed more than 42,000 male doctors, divided the doctors into two groups. One group received a "prudent diet" consisting of vegetables, fruit, fish, poultry, and whole grains. The other group was given the "Western" diet that we know as the Standard American Diet, consisting of red meat, processed meat, French fries, high-fat dairy products, refined grains, and sweets and desserts. Doctors who ate the Western diet carried a fifty- percent increased risk for developing type 2 diabetes. Combine the Western diet with a sedentary lifestyle, and the risk nearly doubled.

CONSEQUENCES OF TYPE 2 DIABETES

Uncontrolled blood sugar levels for prolonged periods can result in serious complications such as nephropathy (kidney disease), neuropathy (nerve damage), retinopathy (vision damage), amputations, and heart disease. Up to forty percent of diabetics will develop related complications.

Regulating blood sugar and insulin levels, keeping within a healthy weight range, and following the diet plan provided in Chapter 10 can help prevent the complications associated with diabetes.

MANAGING DIABETES

More than any other disease or disorder, diabetes is associated with diet. Therefore the management of diabetes relies heavily on what we eat. Food turns into glucose in the blood. The goal for type 2 diabetes is to achieve normal blood sugar levels, between 4 mmol/L (70 mg/dL) and 7 mmol/L (110 mg/dL). This is accomplished by properly balancing diet, exercise, medications, or insulin.

Chapter 10 provides an eating plan to help you achieve long-term successful fat reduction, control inflammation and insulin resistance, and prevent metabolic syndrome, type 2 diabetes, and cardiovascular disease. The program is based on simple concepts—eat fewer calories than you burn, choose only those foods that your body can burn, eat five to six small meals per day, control portion sizes, balance your food groups (low-glycemic carbohydrates, protein at every meal, polyunsaturated fats), and exercise. At the end of the book you will find information on natural supplements that can give you a jump-start. The metabolic syndrome diet plan provided in this book will improve your body's metabolism and increase the sensitivity of the body cells to insulin—both of which are essential to preventing metabolic syndrome.

WHAT YOU HAVE LEARNED IN THIS CHAPTER

- Insulin resistance is the root cause of metabolic syndrome.
- Insulin triggers fat storage, leading to obesity, a prime risk factor for type 2 diabetes.
- Insulin resistance is essentially diabetes. You need to control your insulin levels to prevent many of today's chronic diseases, including obesity, type 2 diabetes, and cardiovascular disease.

In the next chapter we will take a more detailed look at how inflammation can lead to insulin resistance and metabolic syndrome.

Chapter 8

FIRES WITHIN

What is the relationship between insulin resistance, diabetes, obesity, and heart attacks? Although the problem is less obvious than the obesity epidemic, North Americans are also suffering from the inflammation epidemic. Most of us experience inflammation from time to time, the acute kind that occurs when we cut a finger and the area swells and becomes sensitive to the touch. However, inflammation is probably one of the least talked about but most important risk factors for metabolic syndrome. As mentioned in Chapter 7, the kind of inflammation related to metabolic syndrome is chronic, not inflammation we can see, but invisible inflammation throughout our bodies. Every disease has some type of inflammatory component to it, whether it is obesity, diabetes, heart disease, depression, irritable bowel syndrome, autoimmune diseases like arthritis, fibromyalgia, cancer, allergies, or asthma. Even the natural process of aging can be accelerated. But what causes all this inflammation?

New research confirms that obesity is a primary cause of inflammation. In other words, fat cells trigger inflammation. Losing excess body fat will be a key component in your lifelong struggle against inflammation. Inflammation is the smoking gun that links excess body fat to today's epidemic rise in insulin resistance and metabolic syndrome.

Treatment and control of inflammation may reduce the risk of insulin resistance and thereby prevent metabolic syndrome and other related diseases.

INFLAMMATION: A NECESSARY EVIL

Your body has its own defense system—the immune system, which is an integrated network of cells that protects the body. It is a highly specialized frontline defense that identifies, remembers, attacks, and destroys disease-causing invaders and infected cells. Essentially the immune system is our bodies' means of surveillance, intended to protect us from disease by searching out and destroying any health-damaging agents. When it functions optimally, the immune system is a powerful protector. Few viruses, bacteria, fungi, or parasites are allowed to set up house and wreak havoc when the immune system is operating at its peak. If the immune system is not protected, it will turn on itself and destroy healthy cells or fail in the face of a viral or bacterial onslaught. Part of the immune system's frontline defense is a process called inflammation.

When inflammation occurs, chemicals from the body's white blood cells are released into the blood or affected tissues to protect us from foreign substances. This release of chemicals increases the blood flow to the area of injury or infection and may result in redness and warmth. Some of the chemicals cause a leak of fluid into the tissues, resulting in swelling. This protective process may stimulate nerves and cause pain.

It is easy to think of inflammation as always being the very thing we should avoid. However, inflammation is a necessary response; the problem is when we have too much of a good thing. There are times when our inflammatory responses go awry and become deregulated. In fact, inflammation can harm the very thing it is meant to heal.

The destructive side of inflammation has long been evident in many of the diseases people are suffering from today. Dr. Floyd Chilton, author of *The Inflammation Nation*, gives a very detailed account of this inflammatory epidemic. The statistics are as mind-boggling as those related to the obesity epidemic. Inflammation is all around us:

- One in three Americans suffers from arthritis.
- Sixty-four million people have heart disease, which is now seen as an inflammatory condition.
- Fifty million Americans suffer from allergies.
- Twenty million have asthma.

Many of these inflammatory conditions are painful and debilitating and can destroy quality of life. At the center of inflammation is the standard American diet.

In Chapter 2, we learned that early humans obtained most of their food from vegetables, fruis, and lean, high-quality meats. Now our carbohydrates are of the refined variety, made mainly from highly processed flours and sugars. These high-caloric foods provide empty calories. Our meat supply has also drastically changed because of the shift in the way we feed our cattle—from grass-fed to grain-fed. Feeding cattle and other animals a grain-based diet high in corn has resulted in meat, eggs, and poultry loaded with pro-inflammatory fats, like arachidonic acid. Compare early humans' diets to our diet today. Do you think our ancestors had drive-through restaurants back then? Not a chance. If asked about the fastest, quickest food available to us, most people would answer drive-through, take-out, or fast food, but in fact, it is raw fruits and vegetables. It has never ceased to amaze me how people will spend thirty minutes sitting in a drive-through line to get food for their families when a meal of raw fruits, vegetables, and other high-quality proteins could be prepared in much less time. This change in our diet has had a massive impact on the diseases we are experiencing today.

FATS AND INFLAMMATION

The saying "You are what you eat" is true when it comes to the food we eat, inflammation, and the obesity epidemic. What most of us don't realize is that every time we sit down to eat a meal, we may be giving ourselves a plate full of inflammation.

The foods we eat play an important role in how we feel. Loading up on junk foods and fast foods tends to make us feel worse due to the unhealthy fats that are used in the cooking processes. Dietary fats can influence the degree of inflammation. Trans fats, namely hydrogenated oils, some margarines, French fries, and other fried foods are pro-inflammatory. In a Harvard study, trans fatty acids were linked to greater inflammation in overweight women. Saturated fats in red meats and full-fat dairy foods are contributors to chronic inflammation, as well. Chapter 3 showed us that eating too many foods rich in omega-6 fatty acids (especially vegetable oils such as corn, safflower, and sunflower) appears to promote inflammation.

On the other hand, omega-3 fats exert anti-inflammatory effects. Diets with lower amounts of omega-3 fats result in less production of pro-inflammatory prostaglandins (hormones). The best omega-3 sources are fatty fish such as salmon, sardines, mackerel, herring, and tuna, as well as fish-oil supplements. Other omega-3 contributors include ground flax, flax seed oil, walnuts and, to a limited degree, green leafy vegetables. Dietary monounsaturated fats (olive oil and macadamia nut oil) also decrease inflammation.

Why are fats so closely related to inflammation? Prostaglandins, substances that increase inflammation, are the primary culprits. The prostaglandins are hormones produced from fatty acids that are directly related to inflammation and pain. Pro-inflammatory prostaglandins are produced from the plethora of the omega-6 vegetable oils that are consumed in the North American diet. Leukotrienes are also inflammatory messenger that can be released by consuming certain types of fats. There are many other types of inflammatory messengers, but the prostaglandins and leukotrienes are the central players involved in the pain and inflammatory pathways. For example, our bodies seem to increase COX-2 levels (chemicals responsible for the production of inflammation) when omega-6 fats greatly exceed omega-3 fats in the foods we eat. Eating more foods with omega-3 fats and lowering consumption of omega-6 fats might make COX-2 less active. For more information on the metabolic pathway and the production of prostaglandins, see Chapter 3, Figures 3.2 and 3.3.

CARBOHYDRATES AND INFLAMMATION

Excessive consumption of sugars and refined starchy carbohydrates such as white flour wreak havoc on the waistline and can also make inflammation worse. Foods that spike blood sugar spur inflammation. In a Harvard study, women who ate foods with the highest glycemic load (see Chapter 4) had nearly twice as much inflammation as other women.

A research study published in the *American Journal of Clinical Nutrition* looked at participants from the Nurses' Health Studies, including 656 women with confirmed type 2 diabetes and 694 controls. Frequent consumption of sugar-sweetened soft drinks, refined grains, diet soft drinks, processed meat and infrequent intake of wine, coffee, and cruciferous and yellow vegetables were associated with an increased risk of type 2 diabetes. The researchers concluded that the dietary pattern identified in the study (too many simple carbohydrates) may increase chronic inflammation and raise the risk of developing type 2 diabetes.

Just as choosing the right fats is important in controlling inflammation, so is choosing the right carbohydrates. There is a complex interaction between the messengers of inflammation and blood sugar levels. This means there is a relationship between the kinds of carbohydrates we consume and inflammation. You need to avoid anything that causes glucose and insulin levels to spike dramatically, which is what happens if you eat too many refined carbohydrates. To avoid inflammation caused by carbohydrates, follow the advice in Chapter 4: consume only low-GI carbohydrates.

THE OBESITY-INFLAMMATION CONNECTION

Inflammation and obesity are intertwined, and diet is a common denominator. With 63% of the population being overweight, we will see an increase in the number of people with inflammatory diseases.

Obesity may be linked to a higher risk of metabolic syndrome in part because of inflammation. Research suggests that the body's fat cells produce cytokines, proteins that raise inflammation. As the size of fat cells increases, so does inflammation. In one study, one measure of inflammation increased by more than fifty percent in obese women whose fat was mainly in their hips and thighs (pear-shaped). In obese women with significant waistline fat (apple-shaped) the increase was more than four hundred percent.

In a recent Italian study, obese women were able to significantly lower their cytokine levels by losing ten percent of their body fat.

Obesity is associated with a state of chronic, low-grade inflammation, and alterations in fat mass are associated with changes in energy intake and storage, insulin sensitivity, and metabolism.

In the *Journal of Clinical Investigation* two studies reported that obese fatty tissue is characterized by an influx of macrophages, which are an important source of inflammation in fat tissue. The body mass index and average fat cell size were significant predictors of macrophages in fat tissue. The study suggested that obesity-related insulin resistance is, at least in part, a chronic inflammatory disease initiated in fat tissue.

Another theory explaining the perils of having excess fat cells is that it taxes the immune system because the body views the fat cells as "foreign invaders." To fight off the invaders, the body turns on the inflammatory response and keeps it on.

THE HEART DISEASE-INFLAMMATION CONNECTION

Why does extra fat around the waist increase the risk of heart disease? A study published in the *American Journal of Physiology* suggests that inflammation may be the key. Inflammation is a bigger threat to your heart than cholesterol. The risk of heart attack jumped 300 percent in women with high blood vessel inflammation, but only 40 percent in women with high bad-type LDL cholesterol, according to a study from Harvard. Men with the most severe inflammation had three times the odds of dying from a heart attack as men with the least inflammation.

The link between obesity and heart disease is not completely understood, yet study data suggest that inflammatory proteins produced by fat itself may play a role. One study evaluated whether inflammatory proteins produced by fat are linked to risk factors for heart disease, including high blood pressure, high cholesterol, and how the body responds to insulin. The research is based on a new idea in medicine that fat is an organ that produces proteins and hormones that affect metabolism and health.

The researchers studied two proteins that promote inflammation (interleukin 6 and tumor necrosis factor alpha) and a protein that promotes blood clots (plasminogen activator inhibitor 1). These proteins are all manufactured by fat tissue and involved in atherosclerosis, the buildup of fatty deposits in the linings of blood vessels. The scientists also looked at two good proteins: leptin, which regulates energy metabolism, and adiponectin, which has anti-inflammatory effects.

The study included twenty postmenopausal women fifty to seventy years old who were overweight or obese and had waists larger than thirty-five inches. Women in this age group are at increased risk for metabolic syndrome, which increases the risk for heart disease.

In fifteen study participants who did not have diabetes, higher levels of the bad proteins interleukin 6 and tumor necrosis factor alpha were associated with a lower ability to respond to insulin and use glucose. On the other hand, higher levels of the good protein adiponectin were associated with an increased ability to use glucose. Eight women who were diagnosed with metabolic syndrome and had multiple risk factors for heart disease had levels of adiponectin that were thirty-two percent lower than the twelve women who didn't have the disorder. This suggests that low production of adiponectin in subcutaneous fat is linked with an elevated risk of heart disease.

The findings are significant because of the prevalence of both heart disease and obesity in the United States. Heart disease is the number-one killer in the United States and Canada, causing about 79,000 more deaths per year than the next five leading causes of death combined.

Researchers have begun to test whether diet and exercise will affect levels of the proteins. Scientists already know that weight loss and physical activity can reduce inflammation, but they don't know if this happens because the production of inflammatory proteins by fat tissue is reduced.

A primary goal for heart attack prevention should be to keep inflammation to a minimum.

C-REACTIVE PROTEIN

Cardiologists have found a new way to assess a person's risk of atherosclerosis (hardening of the arteries): they measure a substance in the blood called C-reactive protein (CRP), a marker of inflammatory activity. Two large studies—one in men and one in women—have demonstrated that the higher a person's C-reactive protein level, the greater the risk of a heart attack or stroke.

Researchers say CRP has previously been found only in the liver or within blood vessel walls, where it is produced in response to inflammatory triggers. But new results suggest that body fat may also be capable of producing the protein, which has been linked to an increased risk of heart disease and stroke. This may help explain why overweight people face a higher risk of heart disease and stroke as well as shed new light on the link between inflammation and these disorders.

In a new study published in the *Journal of the American College of Cardiology*, researchers looked at whether body fat cells could produce C-reactive protein under a variety of conditions in the lab.

The results showed that fat cells produced inflammatory cytokines, which resulted in inflammation and then triggered the production of high levels of C-reactive protein.

In addition, researchers found that resistan, a hormone produced by body fat cells associated with diabetes and insulin resistance, also triggered the production of CRP.

If fat cells by themselves produce inflammatory signals that trigger cells to produce CRPs, and if CRPs also produce biological effects on vascular walls, that could explain the higher risk of cardiovascular disease.

TYPE 2 DIABETES-INFLAMMATION CONNECTION

Insulin resistance is the predominant mechanism associated with type 2 diabetes and is also central to the development of metabolic syndrome. In the last several years there has been a growing body of evidence that chronic low-grade inflammation is a potential cause of insulin resistance and type 2 diabetes. This information ties in with new data that heart disease, the main complication of insulin resistance and diabetes, has a major inflammatory component as well.

Abnormal levels of inflammatory markers such as CRP and prothrombotic markers like plasminogen activator inhibitor-1 (PAI-1) have been reported in insulin-resistant subjects and may contribute to the increased cardiovascular events in this population in combination with abnormal cholesterol and high blood pressure. Inflammation may also be important in diabetes. Elevated CRP levels are associated with a higher-than-average risk of developing Type 2 diabetes.

In diabetes, excess body fat—a major risk factor for the disease—may be part of the inflammatory picture. Fat cells produce cytokines, the proteins that promote inflammation. Studies have shown that people who develop type 2 diabetes have relatively high levels of these cytokines. Researchers think the cytokines may interfere with the body's ability to use its own insulin, thus bringing on diabetes.

Data from the Third National Health and Nutrition Examination Survey of 1988–1993 (NHANES III) further support the hypothesis that insulin resistance and inflammation are related. This study was carried out in nearly 10,000 U.S. adults twenty years or older. The results show a strong relation between serum ferritin levels—a marker of inflammation—and impaired fasting glucose and newly diagnosed diabetes, conditions characterized by insulin resistance.

ANTI-INFLAMMATORY LIFESTYLE

The rise of obesity, insulin resistance, diabetes, and heart disease in the past several decades has paralleled a dramatic change in the Western lifestyle. A study followed 42,000 male health professionals for more than twelve years. Researchers found that men who consumed a typical Western diet—including lots of red and processed meat, high-fat dairy products, French fries, and refined grains, sweets, desserts, high-sugar drinks, and other rapidly absorbed, high-glycemic index carbohydrates—were more likely to develop diabetes than those whose diets centered on vegetables, fish, and poultry, more fiber, higher intakes of protein, and less refined and more slowly absorbed, low-glycemic carbohydrates. The twenty percent of men who followed the typical Western diet were sixty percent more likely to develop diabetes than the twenty percent who followed a healthier diet. The combination of the Western diet with a low level of physical activity or obesity was associated with a higher risk of type 2 diabetes.

An explanation of this study is that the Western diet enhances inflammation, which gives rise to insulin resistance. Dietary glycemic index and load are predictors of type 2 diabetes and of heart disease risk factors. In a study of 244 healthy, middle-aged women, a higher dietary glycemic load was directly related to CRP levels. These data suggest that eating too many rapidly absorbed carbohydrates increases risk of heart disease and diabetes through inflammatory mediators.

Also, the increased prevalence of diabetes has paralleled an increased consumption of omega-6 fatty acids and trans fats. This has risen as fats from fish, wild game, and leaves were replaced by the consumption of linoleic acid-rich oils from seeds. Changes in feeding poultry and livestock have also altered the omega-6 to omega-3 ratio of animal protein. This imbalance leads to high levels of pro-inflammatory omega-6s and the production of inflammatory mediators.

Since lack of exercise leads to obesity, and obesity is an inflammatory condition, increased exercise may improve markers of inflammation. Level of fitness is a strong predictor of diabetes. For example, in a study of 25,000 men followed for an average of eight years, the fatter the men, the greater the mortality risk. However, when categorized according to level of cardiovascular fitness (treadmill performance), weight did not matter as much as fitness levels. Those who were physically fit, but obese, had a lower risk of dying than unfit men of normal weight. Fit men were found to have greater longevity than unfit men regardless of body composition. Patients with diabetes and a high fitness level had a seventy percent lower risk of dying compared to those who were not fit. An explanation of these findings is that exercise not only improves blood sugar levels, blood pressure, cholesterol, and triglycerides and reduces body fat, but it also improves insulin sensitivity and reduces inflammatory markers like CRP.

Therefore, lifestyle changes—which are the basis for the treatment for insulin resistance, diabetes, and heart disease—also mediate their effects in part through anti-inflammatory pathways. Identify foods to which you have an allergy or sensitivity, Here is a list of pro-inflammatory foods to avoid:

- Red meats from corn-fed, antibiotic/hormone-laden animals
- Saturated fats such as lard and other meat fats
- Fried foods
- Partially hydrogenated fats (trans fats) found in margarines, chips, candies, cereals, and baked goods—eliminate all trans fats
- Refined cooking oils from corn, safflower, sunflower, or soy
- Soft drinks (both sugar and diet varieties)
- Excess sugar (from heavily processed sources such as candy and from naturally occurring sources such as fruit juice)

Eat organic whenever possible. Anti-inflammatory foods include:

- Foods high in omega-3s, especially cold-water, wild-caught fish (or fish oil supplements)
- Raw nuts and seeds (especially pecans, almonds, walnuts, and flax seeds)
- Dark green vegetables (especially kale, seaweed, and greens)
- Antioxidants in supplement form (especially vitamins C and E and quercitin)
- Zinc taken in supplement form, which assists healing and reduces inflammation
- Extra-virgin olive oil, coconut oil, macadamia nut oil

To limit the inflammation resulting from our food supply, we need to make numerous changes in our diet.

Essential Fatty Acids

The right type of fats in our diets will impact pain and inflammation in a positive way. Omega-3 oils in cold-water oily fish, walnuts, and flax seeds will reduce inflammation. It is beneficial to supplement your diet with a high-quality fish oil capsule (I recommend one gram of omega-3s per day; check the label to achieve the appropriate dose). Gamma linolenic acid (GLA) from borage and evening primrose oil is another potent anti-inflammatory fat. This fat is limited in our food supply, so a supplement must be taken. To reduce inflammation, aim for one gram of GLA per day. Olive oil will help decrease inflammation. See Chapter 12 for further supplement suggestions.

Protein

Eat lean meats and poultry that are free-range, organic and not corn-fed (grass-fed preferably). Avoid or limit your intake of cow's milk products. Good protein choices include lean poultry, turkey, and oily fish such as tuna, salmon, and halibut. Omega-3 eggs are a great source of protein and have higher levels of omega-3 oils than regular eggs. Walnuts, almonds, and legumes round out the list of healthy anti-inflammatory proteins. Incorporating whey protein supplements is also recommended. Follow the dietary advice given in Chapter 10 by incorporating two whey protein shakes (25 grams of protein each) per day.

Carbohydrates

Eat a wide variety of vegetables (the darker and deeper the color, the better). Avoid sugar altogether and incorporate only low-glycemic index carbohydrates (see Chapter 4 for suggestions). Choose green leafy vegetables, green and brightly colored vegetables, and fresh fruits. Berries are a great choice. Apples and red onions are great sources of quercetin, which has strong anti-inflammatory properties.

WHAT YOU HAVE LEARNED IN THIS CHAPTER

• Inflammation is all around us—the primary culprit is the standard American diet. Some inflammation is necessary; the problem is we have too much of a good thing.
• Inflammation leads to insulin resistance, obesity, metabolic syndrome, type 2 diabetes, and heart disease.
• Dietary and lifestyle changes are paramount in controlling inflammation.

In the next chapter we will learn how metabolic syndrome, and primarily insulin resistance, lead to cardiovascular disease.

Chapter 9

HAVE A HEALTHY HEART

Look down the aisles at your neighborhood grocery store and you will see why about one out of every four people has the cluster of disorders dubbed metabolic syndrome. Ninety percent of the products on the supermarket shelves are highly processed foods that are rich in unhealthy fats, loaded with sugar, and depleted of fiber. Combine these foods with lifestyles marked by inactivity, sleep deprivation, and stress, and you create a constellation of physiological phenomena that includes abdominal obesity, low levels of beneficial high-density lipoprotein (HDL), high levels of harmful triglycerides, elevated blood sugar, and high blood pressure. So many adults in the United States and Canada meet the diagnostic criteria for metabolic syndrome that the total number now afflicted nearly equals the number of baby boomers.

"Heart disease" is a term that applies to many diseases or injuries to the cardiovascular system, which includes the heart, the blood vessels of the heart, and the system of blood vessels—veins and arteries—throughout the body and within the brain. One in four Canadians has some form of heart disease—about eight million people. About sixty million Americans suffer from heart disease, and 2,600 people die from it each day. More than two hundred risk factors have been identified for heart disease; common risk factors include high stress, high cholesterol, high blood pressure, high triglycerides, a sedentary lifestyle, smoking, poor diet, obesity, diabetes, and of course metabolic syndrome.

Millions of people are suffering from metabolic syndrome—most don't even know they have it, yet it carries a twofold risk of heart disease and a five times greater chance of developing type 2 diabetes. Metabolic syndrome will overtake cigarette smoking as the number-one risk factor for heart disease among the U.S. population. During the groundbreaking Framingham Heart Study, when the link between high cholesterol and heart attack risk became clear, researchers noticed a certain group of people with low LDL (bad cholesterol) levels who nevertheless had a high risk of heart disease. Why? The study further revealed a cluster of heart disease risk factors, which we now call metabolic syndrome: high levels of insulin and blood sugar, high triglyceride levels, low HDL (good cholesterol), small and dense LDL particles (the kind more likely to burrow into artery walls and cause plaque), high blood pressure, and being overweight.

The seriousness of metabolic syndrome as a heart disease risk factor is clear. In a study of 4,483 people, those with metabolic syndrome were three times more likely to have coronary heart disease, a stroke, or heart attack than those without the syndrome. Another study found that for every thirty-percent increase in insulin production there is a seventy-percent increase in the risk of heart disease over a five-year period. Investigators from the National Health and Nutrition Examination Survey II noted that the metabolic syndrome more strongly predicted coronary heart, cardiovascular, and total mortality than its individual components.

In another study researchers followed 1,209 men ages 42 to 60 who were free from heart disease, cancer, or diabetes for more than eleven years to assess the link between metabolic syndrome and heart disease and death. The study found that men with metabolic syndrome, as defined by the World Health Organization (see Chapter 1), were 2.9 to 3.3 times more likely to die from coronary heart disease. They also found that those with metabolic syndrome, as defined by the National Cholesterol Education

Program (NCEP), were 2.9 to 4.2 times more likely to die from coronary heart disease.

BLOOD MARKERS DEFINED

Cholesterol Crazy

Cholesterol is one of the most misunderstood subjects in nutrition. It is a heart disease risk factor that receives more attention than any other heart-related factor. We are usually left with the impression that if we got rid of the cholesterol from our food—that is, if we stopped eating butter, bacon, and eggs—our cholesterol levels would go down. However, eighty percent of cholesterol comes from our liver. Cholesterol is found within the bloodstream and in every cell in our body. Cholesterol is used to form cell membranes and is needed to produce sex hormones as well as to manufacture vitamin D.

Transporters

Cholesterol is transported in the blood in various protein components known as lipoproteins, including low-density lipoproteins (LDL), high-density lipoproteins (HDL), intermediate-density lipoproteins (IDL), and very low-density lipoproteins (VLDL). These transport proteins vary in their effects in the body. If too much LDL cholesterol circulates in the blood, it can slowly build up on the walls of the arteries, where it can form plaque, a thick, hard deposit that can clog arteries. This condition is known as atherosclerosis (hardening of the arteries). LDL cholesterol has become known as our "bad" cholesterol because of what it does inside arteries. It takes cholesterol to our circulatory system, which can then lead to clots and heart attacks. In metabolic syndrome, LDL levels are often not elevated, however. If their particle size is measured, the LDL particles tend to be smaller and denser, which increases their potential for forming plaques on the artery walls, further leading to heart attacks. The American Heart Association recommends that our LDL cholesterol should be less than 2.6 mmol/L (100 mg/dL).

How to Lower LDL Levels:

- If you are in the moderate to high LDL cholesterol range, that is, 3.3 mmol/L (130 mg/dL) or higher if you have coronary heart disease or 4.9 mmol/L (190 mg/dL) if you are without coronary heart disease, then medication may be required initially to bring levels down to a safe range.
- Numerous studies show that lifestyle changes such as exercise, smoking cessation, weight loss, and following a healthy diet can reduce cholesterol levels and thus the risk of heart disease.
- Eat cholesterol-lowering foods. These include avocadoes, almonds, olive oil, soybeans, garlic, shiitake mushrooms, chili peppers, oat bran, beans (kidney, pinto, black, navy), onions, fatty fish, and flax seeds.
- Take natural supplements (see Chapter 12).

On the other hand, research shows that HDL, also known as our "good" cholesterol, tends to carry the cholesterol it contains from the arteries back to the liver for disposal. HDL acts like a bottom feeder in a fish tank. It cleans off the walls of blood vessels, thus removing the excess LDL cholesterol. The HDL then carries this cholesterol to the liver where it is processed. Some experts believe that HDL removes excess cholesterol from plaques and therefore slows their growth. A high HDL level protects against heart disease, whereas a low HDL level is a component of metabolic syndrome and increases the risk of heart disease. Even small increases in HDL cholesterol reduce the frequency of heart attacks. For each 0.03 mmol/L (1 mg/dL) or 1% increase in HDL cholesterol there is a two to four percent reduction in the risk of coronary heart disease.

Those with metabolic syndrome will have elevated total cholesterol; the bad usually remains within normal levels, and the good cholesterol decreases. The decreasing good cholesterol increases the ratio between LDL and HDL, and a high LDL to HDL ratio is another risk factor associated with cardiovascular disease.

To Increase HDL Levels:

- Regular cardio exercise (aerobic exercise) that burns between 1,200 and 1,500 calories each week can have dramatic results.
- By losing ten pounds of excess weight (fat) you will see significant increases in your HDL cholesterol.
- If you smoke, quit—cigarettes decrease HDL cholesterol levels. According to a study at Vanderbilt, within just one week of quitting smoking, HDL levels rose by seven points.
- Lower carbohydrate intake by avoiding sugar, flour, white potatoes, and white rice. Studies prove that HDL levels drop dramatically when blood sugar is spiked by carbohydrates.
- Take natural supplements (see Chapter 12).

Triglycerides

Triglycerides are a storage form of fat. They come from the food we eat and from the foods produced by the body. Fatty acids get stored as triglycerides, as do excess sugars/refined carbohydrates. Our bodies have a limited capacity to utilize sugar, so once it reaches that capacity, the sugar gets converted into fat and stored as a triglyceride. During the low-fat, no-fat diet craze in the 1980s and 1990s, many people were eating low-fat food products that were loaded with simple sugars; during this time the triglyceride levels soared through the roof. This is why we need to eat only those carbohydrates that can be burned. Elevated triglyceride levels are positively associated with an increased risk of heart disease, and triglycerides greater than 1.7 mmol/L (150 mg/dL) are a component of metabolic syndrome.

When looking at markers for metabolic syndrome, it makes sense to consider the effects of low HDL cholesterol and high triglyceride levels. The science shows that each of these factors is related to greater risk of coronary heart disease. People with high triglycerides often have low HDL levels and small, dense LDL particles. Many genetic and environmental influences are related to HDL and triglycerides. For example, low HDL levels are found in cigarette smokers, obese persons, and inactive individuals. A low HDL level—1.0 mmol/L (<40 mg/dL) in men and 1.3 mmol/L (<50 mg/dL) in women—is one of the diagnosing criteria for metabolic syndrome.

To understand why these lipid changes occur in patients with insulin resistance, it is important to remember the role insulin has in the metabolism of free fatty acids (FFAs) and the production of triglycerides. In insulin resistance, there is an increase in FFA released from fat cells. This increase causes circulating levels of FFA to rise, which stimulates the production of triglyceride-rich HDL and LDL particles. The increase in triglycerides in lipid particles changes their metabolism. Triglyceride-rich HDL particles are dissolved more rapidly, and HDL levels fall, a negative consequence. The triglyceride-enriched LDL particles are subject to further breakdown, which gives rise to the formation of small, dense LDL particles. The low HDL levels and the increased formation of the small, dense LDL particles are strongly related to increasing atherosclerosis (hardening of the arteries), and account for some of the increase in cardiovascular disease risk that occurs in insulin-resistant or metabolic syndrome individuals.

To Lower your Triglyceride Levels:

- Cut back on simple sugars like juices, soda, pastries, pies, candy, cookies, and sweet desserts.
- Decrease or eliminate alcohol, as excessive alcohol contributes to high triglyceride levels.
- Reduce carbohydrate-containing foods such as bread, pasta, white rice, and white flour. Some people could be sensitive to such foods; eating them could lead to elevated triglycerides. Instead, choose low- and medium-glycemic index carbohydrates like whole-wheat pasta, brown rice, barley, and oats in moderation.
- Obesity is shown as a major cause of high triglycerides. If you are overweight, lose weight with regular exercise and by reducing totally calorie intake.
- Take natural supplements (see Chapter 12).

Recommended Cholesterol Levels (American Heart Association and National Cholesterol Education Program)

Total Cholesterol: Less than 200 mg/dL (5.1 mmol/L)
LDL Cholesterol: Less than 100 mg/dL (2.56 mmol/L)
HDL Cholesterol: Women>50 mg/dL (1.3 mmol/L)
                        Men >40 mg/dL (1.0 mmol/L)
Triglycerides: Less than 150 mg/dL (1.7 mmol/L)

HIGH BLOOD PRESSURE: A TWENTY-FIRST CENTURY EPIDEMIC

High blood pressure, or hypertension, means high pressure in the arteries. The arteries are the vessels that carry blood from the pumping heart to all the tissues and organs of the body. Normal blood pressure is below 120/80; blood pressure between 120/80 and 139/89 is called "pre-hypertension," and a blood pressure of 140/90 or above is considered high blood pressure. The systolic blood pressure, which is the first number, is the pressure in the arteries as the heart contracts and pumps blood into the arteries. The diastolic pressure, which is the second number, is the pressure in the arteries as the heart relaxes after the contraction. The diastolic pressure, therefore, reflects the minimum pressure to which the arteries are exposed.

If you have hypertension, there is a high likelihood that you have at least some of the characteristics of metabolic syndrome. In fact, the association is so strong that hypertension should be regarded as a significant risk factor for future diabetes.

Moreover, the estimate of 47 million U.S. adults with metabolic syndrome is based on the rather lax definition of hypertension as a blood pressure greater than 140/90 mm/Hg. Many truly hypertensive people will be uncounted using this guideline. It is also clear that blood pressure begins to affect mortality rates at levels above 115 mm/Hg. Most people are shocked when they hear this, having been accustomed to hypertension guidelines specifying levels of 150/90 mm/Hg and higher. To remind ourselves of what optimal blood pressure should be, we need only look at blood pressure levels in primitive cultures that lack access to processed foods and are engaged in physical activity much of the day. People in these cultures, who rarely suffer from cardiovascular disease, have blood pressures of around 90/60 mm/Hg.

High blood pressure increases your chance of getting heart disease and/or kidney disease, and of having a stroke. It is especially dangerous because it often has no warning signs or symptoms. Regardless of race, age, or gender, anyone can develop high blood pressure. It is estimated that one in every four American adults has high blood pressure.

High blood pressure occurs in up to one-third of those with metabolic syndrome. Insulin resistance has been directly tied to the development of high blood pressure. Obesity and weight gain in middle age are also associated with high blood pressure. Insulin increases the secretion of cortisol, a stress hormone that constricts blood vessels and is strongly associated with heart disease. This fact, along with research showing that reduction of blood pressure to less than 130/85 mm/Hg in people with diabetes and other people at risk for heart disease, has led to the inclusion of high blood pressure in the diagnosis of metabolic syndrome. It is possible that treating insulin resistance will help lower blood pressure.

Stop High Blood Pressure, Address Metabolic Syndrome

Metabolic syndrome is by far the leading trigger for hypertension today. It is also a very correctable cause. Correcting metabolic syndrome can have a tremendous impact on blood pressure. It is important to take steps to keep your blood pressure under control. The treatment goal is blood pressure below 130/85 mm/Hg and lower for people with other conditions, such as diabetes and kidney disease. Adopting healthy lifestyle habits is effective in both preventing and controlling high blood pressure.

The most powerful way to regain control of multifaceted metabolic syndrome and high blood pressure is to lose weight, and there are many ways to do it. People with metabolic syndrome respond especially well to diets that restrict carbohydrates and focus on low-glycemic index foods that slow the release of blood sugar. If you succeed in losing weight, you are very likely to reduce your blood pressure enough (frequently by 10 to 40 mm/Hg systolic).

Treatment for high blood pressure should also focus on reducing salt intake in the diet. A key to healthy eating is choosing foods lower in salt. Most people consume more salt than they need. The current recommendation is to consume less than 2.4 grams (g), or 2,400 milligrams (mg), of sodium a day. That equals 6 grams (about 1 teaspoon) of table salt a day. The 6 grams include *all* salt and sodium consumed, including salt used in cooking, salt that comes with processed/packaged foods, and salt added at the table. According to the Dietary Approaches to Stop Hypertension (DASH) study, people who consumed a diet low in saturated fat and high in carbohydrates experienced a significant reduction in blood pressure, even without weight reduction. The DASH diet emphasizes fruit, vegetables, low-fat dairy products, whole grains, poultry, fish, and nuts, while reducing saturated fat, red meats, sweets, and beverages containing sugar. Reducing sodium intake can further reduce blood pressure or prevent the increase in blood pressure that may accompany aging.

Tips for Reducing Salt in Your Diet

- Buy fresh, plain, frozen or "no salt added" vegetables
- Use fresh poultry, lean meat, or fish rather than canned or processed varieties
- Replace salt with herbs, spices, and other no-sodium seasonings in cooking and at the table
- When available, buy low-sodium, reduced-sodium, or no-salt-added versions of foods
- Cook rice, pasta, and hot cereals without salt. Cut back on instant or flavored rice, pasta, and cereal mixes, which usually have added salt
- Limit consumption of packaged and convenience foods that are high in sodium
- Pass on the salt shaker at the table—let the natural flavor of food come out

---

Other lifestyle factors should also be examined. Limit alcohol consumption. Drinking too much alcohol can raise blood pressure. It also can harm the liver, brain, and heart. Alcoholic drinks also contain calories, which matter if you are trying to lose weight. If you drink alcoholic beverages, have only a moderate amount—one drink a day for women; two drinks a day for men. Twelve ounces of beer or five ounces of wine counts as one drink.

Being physically active is one of the most important steps you can take to prevent or control high blood pressure. Physical activity also helps reduce your risk of heart disease. It doesn't take a lot of effort to become physically active. See Chapter 11 for tips on physical activity.

Smoking injures blood vessel walls and speeds up the process of hardening of the arteries. So even though it does not cause high blood pressure, smoking is bad for anyone, especially those with high blood pressure. Once you quit smoking, your risk of having a heart attack is reduced after the first year, so you have a lot to gain by quitting.

You can take steps to prevent high blood pressure by adopting a healthy lifestyle. These steps include maintaining a healthy weight; being physically active; following a healthy eating plan that emphasizes fruits, vegetables, and low-fat dairy foods; choosing and preparing foods with less salt and sodium; and, if you drink alcoholic beverages, drinking in moderation.

SUGAR AND HEART DISEASE

We have talked extensively about the dangers of too much sugar in our diet. Research confirms that sugar causes heart disease and makes blood platelet cells—the type of cells that form blood clots—stickier and more likely to clump together. Sticky platelets increase the risk of heart disease and stroke. Sugar also increases triglyceride levels (because the sugar our body can't burn is converted into fat, and stored as triglycerides), as well as the LDL to HDL ratio, both of which are significant risk factors for heart disease.

According to researchers at the Johns Hopkins Bloomberg School of Public Health and other institutions, in a study published in the September 2005 issue of *Archives of Internal Medicine*, lowering blood sugar levels could reduce the risk of coronary heart disease in both diabetics and non-diabetics. The researchers found that Hemoglobin A1c (HbA1c), a measure of long-term blood glucose level, predicts heart disease risk in both diabetics and non-diabetics.

The researchers used data from the Atherosclerosis Risk in Communities Study (ARIC) of almost 16,000 people from four states: North Carolina, Mississippi, Maryland, and Minnesota. HbA1c levels were taken from ARIC study participants during clinical examinations from 1990 to 1992. ARIC researchers tracked study participants for ten to twelve years to record coronary heart disease events, hospitalizations, and deaths.

In participants with diabetes, the researchers found a graded association between HbA1c and increasing coronary heart disease risk. Each one percentage-point increase in HbA1c level was associated with a fourteen-percent increase in heart disease risk. According to the study authors, the current target for "good" glycemic control established by the American Diabetes Association is an HbA1c value of less than seven percent. However, the researchers' analyses suggest that heart disease risk begins to increase at values even below seven percent.

Study participants who did not have diabetes but who had "high normal" HbA1c levels (approximately 5 to 6 percent) were at increased risk for heart disease, even after accounting for other factors such as age, cholesterol level, blood pressure, body mass index, and smoking. Non-diabetic persons with HbA1c levels of 6 percent or higher had almost twice as great a risk of heart disease compared to persons with an HbA1c level less than 4.6 percent.

Diabetes Leads to Heart Attacks

About five to ten percent of people with metabolic syndrome will go on to develop type 2 diabetes. Diabetes significantly increases the risk of heart disease. In fact, some eighty percent of people with diabetes eventually die of heart disease. However, you can reduce your chances of developing heart disease by keeping your blood sugar levels in a normal range, between 4 to 7 mmol/L (70 to 110 mg/dL), losing weight (even ten pounds will make a difference), being physically active, and making healthier dietary choices—choosing low-glycemic index carbohydrates, lean, high-quality protein, and healthy fats. Diabetes can contribute to an imbalance between HDL and LDL. And like people with metabolic syndrome, diabetics tend to have smaller, denser LDL particles, which can lead to more plaque. To make matters worse, blood sugar latches onto lipoproteins, and sugar-coated LDL stays in the bloodstream longer than normal LDL, presenting more opportunities for oxidation, which leads to inflammation and triggers heart disease.

Blood sugar also binds to proteins on the surface of the cells, damaging the artery walls. This blood vessel assault is one of the factors that leads to blindness and kidney damage in people with uncontrolled diabetes, and researchers suspect the same forces are at work with coronary heart disease. But since the blood vessels leading to the eyes and kidneys are smaller and more delicate than those leading to the heart, that damage will turn up sooner.

OBESITY AND HEART DISEASE

Obesity is a major risk factor for heart disease. This is alarming when you consider that one out of every three Americans is obese. Recent studies have shown that obesity is linked to 280,000 deaths in the United States each year, making it second only to cigarette smoking as a cause of death.

Being overweight increases your risk of developing high blood pressure. In fact, blood pressure rises as body weight increases. Losing even ten pounds can lower blood pressure, and it has the greatest effect for those who are overweight and already have hypertension.

The Nurses Health Study found that the risk of developing coronary artery disease increased three to four times in women who had a BMI greater than 29. A Finnish study showed that for every one kilogram (2.2 pounds) increase in body weight, the risk of death from coronary artery disease increased by one percent. In patients who have already had a heart attack, obesity is associated with an increased likelihood of a second heart attack.

Overweight and obesity are also risk factors for heart disease. They increase your chance for developing high blood cholesterol and diabetes, two more major risk factors for heart disease.

Until recently the relation between obesity and heart disease was viewed as indirect, that is, through components related to both obesity and coronary heart disease risk, including high blood pressure; abnormal lipids, particularly reductions in HDL cholesterol; and impaired glucose tolerance or non-insulin-dependent diabetes mellitus. Insulin resistance is typically associated with these components. Although most of the components relating obesity to heart disease increase as BMI increases, they also relate to body fat.

C-REACTIVE PROTEIN LEADS TO HEART DISEASE

In Chapter 8 we learned that C-reactive protein (CRP), a protein produced by the liver when arteries become inflamed, is a marker of inflammation. In the Journal of the *American Heart Association*, researchers showed that out of the 14,719 women who participated in the Women's Health Study, 3,597 were diagnosed with metabolic syndrome. Women in the study who had the highest CRP levels were two times more likely to have a cardiovascular event than those who had only metabolic syndrome. This information demonstrates that inflammation is a critical link between the metabolic syndrome, diabetes, and heart disease.

FREE RADICALS AND HEART DISEASE

To understand how free radicals cause heart disease, you have to understand a bit about cells and molecules. The body is made out of many different types of cells. Cells are composed of many different types of molecules. Molecules consist of one or more atoms joined by chemical bonds. The nucleus of an atom is surrounded by a cloud of electrons. These electrons surround the nucleus in pairs, but occasionally an atom loses an electron, leaving the atom with an "unpaired" electron. Such an atom is called a "free radical," and free radicals are very reactive. When cells in the body encounter a free radical, the reactive radical may cause destruction in the cells. According to Dr. Harmon's free radical theory of aging (he was the first to discover this in 1954), cells continuously produce free radicals, and constant free radical damage eventually kills the cells.

Free radicals are a cause of virtually all diseases, including cancer and heart disease. When a free radical comes in contact with LDL cholesterol, it steals an electron from it, thereby oxidizing the cholesterol. Oxidized LDL cholesterol is more likely to be deposited in your arteries and contribute to the formation of plaque. To combat the free radical damage, the body requires antioxidants.

The Disease-Fighting Antioxidants

A diet high in antioxidants may reduce the risk of many diseases, including heart disease and certain cancers. Antioxidants neutralize the free radicals from the body cells and prevent or reduce the damage caused by oxidation. Flavonoids, such as the tea catechins found in green tea, are believed to contribute to the low rates of heart disease in Japan.

Perhaps the most promising and best-studied area in which antioxidants might play a valuable role is heart disease. Research has demonstrated that the circulation of oxidized LDL promotes atherosclerosis, or hardening of the arteries. In vitro (laboratory) studies have shown that the antioxidant vitamin E can counteract some of the effects of oxidized LDL. The U.S. Nurses Health Study and the Health Professionals Follow-up Study both showed a greater than thirty-percent reduction in the risk of heart disease among those who took supplemental vitamin E.

CoQ10 is another antioxidant that has generated considerable excitement in the areas of heart disease treatment and prevention. CoQ10 has also been called vitamin Q because of its essential role. It is found in abundance in heart muscles, and is produced naturally by our bodies. It is a powerful antioxidant that prevents cellular damaged caused by unstable free radicals.

CoQ10 has been researched for many disease conditions, but most compelling is its role in helping the heart. Without adequate levels of this nutrient, the heart muscle can become weaker and less efficient at pumping blood through the body. Those individuals who have heart disease risk factors, such as high cholesterol, and are taking prescribed statin drugs to lower cholesterol especially need to supplement with CoQ10 because statin drugs shut off the production of CoQ10 from the liver.

There are numerous antioxidants that are beneficial for heart health. For more details on antioxidants in supplement form, see Chapter 12.

Sources of Antioxidants

Good sources of antioxidants include:

- **Allium sulphur compounds:** leeks, onions, and garlic
- **Anthocyanins:** eggplant, grapes, and berries
- **Beta-carotene:** pumpkin, mangoes, apricots, carrots, spinach, and parsley
- **Catechins:** red wine and green tea
- **Copper:** seafood, lean meat, milk, and nuts
- **Cryptoxanthins:** red capsicum, pumpkin, and mangoes
- **Flavonoids:** green tea, citrus fruits, red wine, onions, and apples
- **Indoles:** cruciferous vegetables such as broccoli, cabbage, kale, and cauliflower
- **Isoflavonoids:** soybeans, tofu, lentils, peas, and milk
- **Lignans:** sesame seeds, flax seeds, bran, whole grains, and vegetables
- **Lutein:** leafy greens such as spinach, corn
- **Lycopene:** tomatoes, pink grapefruit, and watermelon
- **Manganese:** seafood, lean meat, milk, and nuts
- **Polyphenols:** thyme and oregano
- **Selenium:** seafood, offal, lean meat, and whole grains
- **Vitamin C:** oranges, black currants, kiwifruits, mangoes, broccoli, spinach, capsicum, and strawberries
- **Vitamin E:** vegetable oils such as wheat germ oil, avocadoes, nuts, seeds, and whole grains
- **Zinc:** seafood, lean meat, milk, and nuts
- **Zoochemicals:** red meat, offal and fish; also derived from the plants animals eat

How to Reduce Heart Disease Risk

Dietary and lifestyle interventions are critical to the management of abnormal blood lipids and high blood pressure. The following changes should be considered:

- Reduce saturated fat and trans fats
- Exercise at least 30 minutes per day, 5 times a week (see Chapter 11)
- Reduce salt in your diet
- Increase consumption of antioxidants in food
- Eat fewer simple sugars; focus on low-glycemic index carbohydrates
- Limit alcohol consumption
- Reduce stress
- Use natural supplements such as omega-3 fish oils, and take antioxidants such as CoQ10 and vitamin E (For more information on supplements, see Chapter 12)

WHAT YOU HAVE LEARNED IN THIS CHAPTER

- Metabolic syndrome is a leading cause of heart disease. Those with metabolic syndrome have a twofold risk of developing heart disease.
- Low HDL, elevated LDL and triglycerides, and high blood pressure are components of the metabolic syndrome and significant risk factors for heart disease.
- Lifestyle and dietary changes are critical to controlling risk factors for heart disease.

In the next chapter you will learn how to eat the right types of food to help you lose weight and prevent and control metabolic syndrome components.

Chapter 10

WEIGHT WARS, BE A WISE LOSER:
The Importance of Weight Loss

Weight loss is a key objective in preventing and dealing with metabolic syndrome. All components of the metabolic syndrome are positively affected by weight loss. Even modest weight reductions, in the range of 5 to 10 percent of initial body weight (10 to 20 pounds for a 200-pound person), are associated with significant improvements.

How do you gain weight? If your energy intake (calorie consumption) is greater than your expenditure, you will gain weight. Energy comes from food and is used for metabolic needs and physical activity. The extra energy is then stored as fat. Cutting back on the number of calories you eat per day (smaller portion sizes), changing the balance of food you eat (focus on low-glycemic carbohydrates, dietary fiber, polyunsaturated fats, and high-quality protein), and increasing energy expenditure in the form of physical activity—together these changes provide a bulletproof system that will help you lose weight safely and effectively. I usually recommend losing 2 pounds per week for people up to 175 pounds. If you are heavier you may lose more. A good calculation to remember is:

Eat 500 fewer calories per day = 1 pound of weight loss per week. Combine that with burning 500 calories per day and you will easily lose 2 pounds per week. It is that simple!

THE SKINNY ON FAD DIETS

Atkins, Beverly Hills, Cabbage Soup, Cider Vinegar, Eat Right 4 Your Type, Grapefruit, Ornish, South Beach, Sugar Busters, Zone, and the list goes on and on. I'm sure most of you have heard of them and some of you may have tried them. Did you ever wonder why there are so many fad diets out there? It's because they don't work. Fat diets are a multibillion dollar industry in which the product is marketed to the consumer with magical claims. In many cases, once you go off the diet, not only do you regain the weight lost but you add some extra as well. The diet industry's success is built on our failures.

But why didn't these fad diets help you lose weight or keep the weight off? Fad diets are generally so unrealistic and so unpleasant that they cannot be maintained for the long term. Most of us trying a fad diet will stop eating the diet because it's too restrictive in food choices, boring, expensive, and overall a stressful experience. A recent study published in the *Annals of Internal Medicine* showed there is little evidence to support the use of many commercial weight-loss programs.

However, there is nothing magical about how these diets work. To successfully lose weight is quite simple—energy (calories) in is less than energy (calories) out. You have to burn more than you eat in a day to lose weight.

Healthy eating is about maintaining a balanced diet to ensure that you are getting all the nutrients your body needs. This means consuming an assortment of foods, in the right amounts, from all the food groups. A proper combination of these foods will ensure that your metabolism and appetite remain in a healthy state.

The eating plan I have designed is to teach you about healthy eating and making the proper food choices because a lasting change in your eating habits and activity level will result in weight loss and eventual maintenance of a healthy weight.

DIETARY CHANGES FOR SUCCESSFUL WEIGHT LOSS

Successful weight loss requires that more energy be expended than consumed on a daily basis. Essentially all energy-restricted diets reduce weight and improve blood sugar control. A recent study from the Harvard School of Public Health compared health outcomes from the typical Western diet to those with a more prudent diet similar to the diet our ancestors ate. Data showed that men who consumed a typical Western diet were sixty percent more likely to develop diabetes than those whose diets centered on vegetables, fruits, whole grains, fish, poultry, nuts, and seeds.

Table 10.1: Western Diet vs. Prudent Diet

Western Diet	Prudent Diet
Red meat	Vegetables
Processed meat	Fruit
French fries	Fish
High-fat dairy products	Whole grains and low GI carbohydrates
Refined grains	Poultry
Sweets and desserts	

Source: Adapted from Van Dam RM, Rimm EB, Willett WC, Stampfer MJ, Hu FB. Ann Int Med. 2002;136:201-209

Taking Stock

To discover more about your food and activity habits, answer the following questions:

1. Do you eat fish and poultry at least three times a week?
   ☐ No   ☐ Yes

2. Do you eat breakfast every day?
   ☐ No   ☐ Yes

3. Do you eat whole grains instead of white or refined grains?
   ☐ No   ☐ Yes

4. Do you eat low-fat dairy products whenever you can?
   ☐ No   ☐ Yes

5. Do you avoid all fried foods as much as possible?

☐ No   ☐ Yes

6. Do you eat 3 to 5 meals per day?

☐ No   ☐ Yes

7. Do you eat fast food less than once a week?

☐ No   ☐ Yes

8. Do you pay attention to portion sizes?

☐ No   ☐ Yes

9. Do you follow a healthy eating plan and avoid going on and off diets?

☐ No   ☐ Yes

10. Do you set aside at least 30 minutes, three times a week, for physical activity?

☐ No   ☐ Yes

Your Score: Count up the number of checks you have in column 2 (yes). What was your score? _____

8 to 10 checks: Fantastic! Keep up the good work.

5 to 7 checks: You're on the right track, but its time to start considering some changes.

0 to 4 checks: Uh-oh. Take time now to make some changes.

Tell Me How

The first step is to make small but significant changes from a Western diet to a more prudent (or ancestral) diet, taking into account the information you have learned about low-glycemic carbohydrates, lean, high-quality proteins, and unsaturated fats.

In the beginning this may be as simple as making the switch from white bread to whole-grain bread; from margarine to butter; from eating hamburger two times per week to eating chicken, turkey, and other leaner cuts of meat. If you have been consuming a poor diet for a number of years and have developed obesity, insulin resistance, and metabolic syndrome, the changes you need to make will not happen overnight. Setting reasonable goals for yourself will be the key to successful weight loss. Table 10.2 lists the recommended nutrient breakdown that will help you be successful in your weight loss plan:

Table 10.2: Recommended Nutrient Intake

Nutrient	Recommended Intake
Total Fat	25–30% of total calories
Saturated fat	<7% of total calories
Polyunsaturated fat	Up to 10% of total calories
Monounsaturated fat	Up to 20% of total calories
Carbohydrate	45–50% of total calories
Fiber	25–30 grams/day
Protein	15–20% of total calories
Total Calories	Balance energy intake and expenditure to achieve desirable body weight. Daily energy expenditure should contribute approximately 250–500 calories per day

Food Guide Recommendations

Figure 10.1: Canada's Food Guide to Healthy Eating

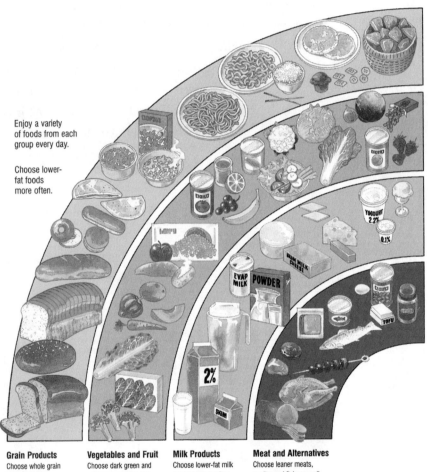

Enjoy a variety
of foods from each
group every day.

Choose lower-
fat foods
more often.

Grain Products
Choose whole grain
and enriched
products more often.

Vegetables and Fruit
Choose dark green and
orange vegetables and
orange fruit more often.

Milk Products
Choose lower-fat milk
products more often.

Meat and Alternatives
Choose leaner meats,
poultry and fish, as well
as dried peas, beans
and lentils more often.

Figure 10.2: USDA Eating Right Pyramid

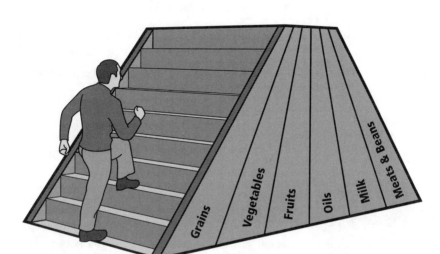

The Canada's Food Guide to Healthy Eating and the USDA Eating Right Pyramid have been criticized in the past for not stressing the importance of quality food choices.

The United States Department of Agriculture and Health Canada feel that bread, cereal, rice, and pasta should make up the bulk of your diet. They recommend a range between five to twelve servings per day, depending on what guide you are following. The Food Guide makes the statement, "Choose whole grains more often." However, that is not clearly understood by the regular consumer, and the food pictures on the Food Guide are white pasta, rice, and bagels. The recommendations for grains do not take into account the glycemic index (GI) of food (see Chapter 4). The GI of food refers to how quickly blood sugar levels rise after eating a certain type of food. Foods with a lower glycemic index will create a slower rise in blood sugar levels, and foods with a higher glycemic index will create a faster rise in blood sugar levels.

Placing the emphasis on carbohydrates is wrong; for the past twenty years we have been told to reduce fat intake and increase carbohydrates. In those years, obesity has more than doubled, and childhood obesity has more than tripled.

The importance of healthy fats is also ignored in the guidelines. Fats help suppress your appetite and don't affect your blood sugar the same way carbohydrates do. That in itself is a major benefit. What people don't realize is that following the governmental food guides will make you fat and insulin resistant, and will increase your likelihood of developing metabolic syndrome, diabetes, and cardiovascular disease.

The Optimal Health Food and Energy Pyramid

The USDA Eating Right Pyramid was updated in April 2005. In the early 1990s there was a lot less emphasis on whole-grain foods than there is today. As well, there is more emphasis on activity now. The new pyramid shows food groups as a series of differently sized colored bands. The bands are different widths to show how much of a particular food group a person should eat each day.

However, most experts agree that the USDA Eating Right Pyramid and Canada's Food Guide are misleading and recommend unhealthy choices. Well-known and respected experts such as Dr. Michael Murray, Dr. Michael Lyon, and Udo Erasmus, as well as many others, have created what they view as healthier recommendations, which take the focus off carbohydrates and more clearly emphasize green foods, healthy oils, fish and lean proteins, nuts, and seeds.

I agree with their recommendations; however, for obesity, insulin resistance, and metabolic syndrome, I am placing an even greater emphasis on protein foods and dairy than they recommend. (See Figure 10.3.) A diet to treat metabolic syndrome aims to improve insulin sensitivity and correct or prevent the associated metabolic and cardiovascular abnormalities. Since most people with metabolic syndrome are overweight, food changes should focus on weight loss, which will improve insulin sensitivity. Research has shown that in most cases a five to ten percent weight reduction is sufficient to induce a significant improvement in insulin resistance. In fact, in many studies, the improvement of insulin sensitivity due to weight reduction is between thirty and sixty percent, which is more than that obtained with insulin-sensitizing drugs.

Figure 10.3: The Optimal Health Food and Energy Pyramid

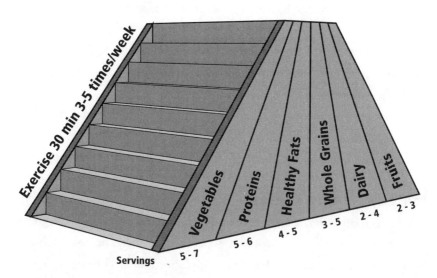

Exercise 30 min 3-5 times/week

Vegetables

Proteins

Healthy Fats

Whole Grains

Dairy

Fruits

Servings   5 - 7   5 - 6   4 - 5   3 - 5   2 - 4   2 - 3

Plus 8 glasses of water
Base Supplement: Whole Food Multiple Vitamin, Omega-3 Fish oil.

Protein Power

Protein is one of the cornerstones to preventing insulin resistance and help-ing with weight loss (see Chapter 5). Protein should be consumed at every meal and snack to help balance carbohydrates and slow down the release of glucose into your bloodstream. To reach your daily requirements of high-quality protein, consume a whey protein shake twice a day.

Eat Dairy, Lose Weight

In my optimal health food recommendations, dairy is also recommended. More and more research is suggesting that the more dairy food consumed, the less likely your chances of metabolic syndrome. While the researchers can-not necessarily explain what is responsible for this association, they say that calcium in the dairy products may have some role to play.

Researchers from the Shaheed Beheshti University of Medical Sciences in Tehran assessed dairy consumption and features of metabolic syndrome in a study of 827 men and women. People consuming the most dairy were more than a third less likely to have a large waist size and almost thirty percent less likely to have high blood pressure. A growing body of research suggests that eating dairy foods may prevent weight gain. They found that the incidence of metabolic syndrome was twenty-nine percent less likely among people with the highest dairy intake.

However, many people are lactose intolerant—that is, they lack the enzyme necessary to digest milk protein or are allergic to milk. If you are lactose intolerant, make sure you are receiving the necessary calcium from a supplement.

It's Easy Being Green

The food group with the largest recommendations is vegetables—the greener the better. Vegetables are nutritional super foods that can help you achieve a healthy weight because they have a low-glycemic index. The veggies are broken down slowly in the body, causing less of a rise in blood sugar levels, less insulin secretion, and ultimately, less fat storage. Vegetables also have a high water and fiber content, which helps promote the feeling of fullness, reduce hunger, and decrease calorie intake.

In a recent study undertaken by Pennsylvania State University, researchers gave forty-two women three cups of low-calorie salad twenty minutes before a meal of pasta to help reduce calorie intake. The results showed that the women ate about one hundred calories less compared to when no salad was served.

Before you eat carbohydrates, try to eat a large portion of leafy greens! Add cucumbers and tomatoes, which count as free vegetables, because they don't affect blood sugar levels.

The food recommendations for optimal health include:

Vegetables (5 to 7 servings): Choose green foods more often. Start lunch and dinner with a green salad. Tomatoes and cucumbers are considered free vegetables, so you can eat as many of these as you like.

Protein (5 to 6 servings, or each time you eat): Lean meat, chicken, turkey, fish, eggs, beans or lentils, whey protein. Eat protein at each meal to balance blood sugar levels. Protein and low-glycemic carbohydrates should be consumed together.

Healthy Fats (4 to 5 servings): Nuts, seeds, avocadoes, fatty fish, oils such as flax seed oil, extra virgin olive oil, macadamia nut oil, butter, and coconut oil. Many healthy fats are also good sources of protein. Focus on the unsaturated fats like the omega-3s and 9s. Supplement with an omega-6 borage or evening primrose oil supplement to get the good omega-6 that is missing in the diet. Avoid using safflower, sunflower, soy, and corn oils, because they contain too much omega-6, linoleic acid, and arachidonic acid, which fuel inflammation.

Whole Grains (3 to 5 servings): Low-glycemic index, fibrous choices only. (See Chapter 4.) Increase fiber consumption to 25 to 30 grams per day. Limit your carbohydrate consumption to what you can actually burn, because what you don't burn will be stored as fat.

Dairy (2 to 4 servings): Choose low-fat, organic dairy foods more often. Try incorporating yogurt, cottage cheese, and kefir into your diet. They are even better than milk, because of their beneficial bacteria. In recent studies, dairy food consumption has been linked to lowered risk of metabolic syndrome. If you can't tolerate dairy, ensure you are taking a calcium supplement to replace the calcium you aren't receiving in your diet.

Fruit (2 to 3 servings): Choose berries and other low-glycemic index fruits. (See Chapter 4.) Fruit plays a much less significant role because of its sugar content. Of the two servings, you should be consuming at least one serving of berries. Avocadoes are an exception, as they are the only fruit that contains the healthy monounsaturated fats, along with vitamins and minerals. So although avocadoes are considered a fruit, they can also be used as part of your healthy fat serving.

See Table 10.3 for appropriate serving sizes.

Other Recommendations:

1. Consume a diet rich in whole, raw foods that have gone through minimal processing. They provide a greater variety of nutrients and bring our diet back to how our ancestors used to eat.

2. Reduce calorie consumption by 500 calories per day to safely lose one pound per week. Combine fewer calories with burning an additional 500 calories per day during exercise, and you can lose two pounds per week. If you weigh more than 175 pounds, it is safe to lose more than two pounds per week.

3. Eat 5 to 6 small meals per day. If you are in the initial phases of weight loss you may want to consider replacing one or two meals per day with a whey protein shake.

4. Avoid starchy or sugary foods—get rid of everything white in your cupboards.

5. Avoid hydrogenated oils (trans fats) and junk foods (high-calorie, low-nutrient foods). Junk foods and processed foods are sent directly to your bloodstream and cause a rapid increase in blood sugar levels and insulin production.

6. Utilize whey protein powders to help stabilize blood sugar levels.

7. Eliminate artificial sweeteners; switch to natural sweeteners like stevia and xylitol.

8. Limit salt intake.

9. Limit alcohol consumption.

10. Exercise daily—try to burn 250 to 500 calories per day. Combine aerobic, strength, and stretching exercises.

11. Drink lots of water—8 glasses per day

12. Supplement with a whole food multivitamin and omega-3 fish oil every day. If you are overweight or if you have insulin resistance, metabolic syndrome, type 2 diabetes, or cardiovascular disease, please see additional supplement recommendations in Chapter 12.

13. Get plenty of sleep. Scientific studies increasingly link lack of sleep to the obesity epidemic.

Portion Distortion

North Americans consume too much food. Cutting back on portion sizes is an easy and effective way to help with weight loss. Recommended portion sizes are not as big as you would think. Here is an example of serving sizes from each group.

Table 10.3: Serving Sizes

One Serving...
Vegetables (5 to 7 servings daily)
1 cup raw greens or salad (about the size of your fist, or what you could hold in one cupped hand)
1/2 cup fresh, frozen, or canned

One Serving...
Protein (5 to 6 servings daily)
50 to 100 g meat, fish, or poultry (about the size of a deck of cards or the palm of your hand)
1/2 to 1 cup beans or lentils
2 tbsp natural peanut butter (about the size of a Ping-Pong ball)
1 to 2 eggs
1/3 to 2/3 can tuna or salmon

One Serving...
Healthy fats (4 to 5 servings daily)
1 tbsp olive oil, macadamia nut oil,
or flax seed oil, or 2 tbsp ground flax seeds
50 g or 2 oz nuts (about a handful)

One Serving...
Whole grains (3 to 5 servings daily)
1/2 cup brown rice or whole wheat pasta (about the size of a light bulb or a small fist)
1/2 cup hot cereal
30 g cold cereal, Bran Flakes for example
1 slice of whole wheat, rye, or multigrain bread

One Serving...
Fruit (2 to 3 servings daily)
One medium sized piece (about the size of a tennis ball)
1/2 cup fresh, frozen, or canned

One Serving...
Dairy (1 to 2 servings daily)
1 cup milk
3/4 cup yogurt
50 g cheese (about the size of two thumbs)

Table 10.4 provides a sample menu meeting these requirements.

Table 10.4: Sample Menu

	Vegetables 5 to 7 servings	Protein 5 to 6 servings	Healthy fats 4 to 5 servings	Whole grains 3 to 5 servings	Fruit 2 to 3 servings	Dairy 2 to 4 servings	Extras
Breakfast			1 tbsp ground flax seeds	3/4 cup oatmeal			
					1/2 cup berries		
						1/2 cup low-fat milk	Coffee
Snack		25 g whey protein mixed with water (counts for 2 servings)					
Lunch	1 cup mixed greens						
	1/2 cup baby carrots	1/2 can tuna packed in water					
		2 oz almonds (counts for 1/2 serving)	also counts for 1 serving				
			1 tbsp olive oil as dressing				
Snack					1/2 cup fresh berries		
		25 g whey protein mixed with water (counts for 2 servings)					

Table 10.4: Sample Menu continued

	Vegetables 5 to 7 servings	Protein 5 to 6 servings	Healthy fats 4 to 5 servings	Whole grains 3 to 5 servings	Fruit 2 to 3 servings	Dairy 2 to 4 servings	Extras
Supper	2 cups mixed greens (add tomatoes, cucumbers). (counts as 2 servings)		1 tbsp of olive oil				
		100 grams grilled chicken breast					
	1 cup steamed broccoli						
				1/2 cup wild rice			
						13/4 cup yogurt	
Snack		1 tbsp ground flax seeds (counts as half serving)	counts as 1 serving				
	5	7.5	5	2	2	2	

Eat More Frequently

As mentioned in Chapter 5, eating five to six smaller meals per day is highly recommended. I recommend breakfast, a protein shake mid-morning, lunch, a protein shake mid-afternoon, dinner, then an optional snack in the evening. Such an eating schedule helps balance blood sugar levels, keeping them even throughout the day, and will prevent peaks and spikes in blood sugar and insulin levels. Maintaining blood sugar and insulin levels is extremely important to help with weight loss and insulin resistance. Including a protein at each meal will also help keep you feeling full and will stabilize your blood glucose levels.

Meal Plans and Meal Replacements

If you are in the beginning phases of weight loss you may want to consider substituting one or two meals a day with a protein shake. In between the protein shakes, you can have snacks containing protein, low-glycemic carbohydrates, vegetables, or berries. Instead of drinking the protein shake between meals, you would use it to replace a meal.

Research has shown that by substituting two meals a day with a protein shake or protein bar and eating a sensible third meal, people lose weight; by replacing one meal a day with a protein shake or meal bar, they maintain their weight. In general, people who drink plenty of water, exercise, and make this dietary change will successfully lose weight.

Studies have shown that a structured eating plan that provides good nutrition and portion control for at least one or two meals a day improves risk factors for the metabolic syndrome (cholesterol, blood sugar, insulin resistance, and blood pressure).

SHOPPING, SHOPPING, SHOPPING

Reading labels and figuring out how to shop in a grocery store are essentials for your new, healthy eating plan. However, making sense of the nutrition information provided on food packaging can be confusing and frustrating.

Here are some tips:

Shop the perimeter of the grocery store. Most grocery stores use the same design. The freshest, healthiest, and most natural foods are on the edges of the stores—in the produce, meat, dairy, and bakery sections. (Skip the pastries and cakes and choose only whole-grain products). Avoid the middle aisles: as a general rule they contain the processed convenience foods. As you have learned, these are the worst foods for your blood sugar levels.

Shop in health food stores whenever possible. They offer more options for healthy eating than do regular grocery stores. However, don't assume that everything you pick up in the health food store will be healthy. The sugary treats and convenience foods may be organic and more nutritious than the snacks in a typical grocery store, but they will still promote insulin resistance. Read the labels carefully.

Label Reading

Figure 10.4: Nutrition Facts Label

Nutrition Facts		
Per 1 Tablespoon (15g)		
Amount		% Daily Value
Calories 100		
Fat 8g		12 %
Saturated 0 g		10 %
+ Trans 1 g		
Cholesterol 3 g		1 %
Sodium 0 mg		0 %
Carbohydrate 0 mg		0 %
Fibre 2 g		8 %
Sugar 0 g		
Protein 4 g		
Vitamin A	0 %	Vitamin C	0 %
Calcium	1 %	Iron	0 %

1. Ingredient lists must be on all packaged foods. The ingredients are listed from most to least by weight. This means that the first item on the list is present in the largest amount. Be aware of different names for similar ingredients. For example, sugar, syrup, molasses, glucose, fructose, and other words ending in "ose" are all forms of sugar.

2. Nutrition claims often appear on food labels to focus attention on a certain feature of the food. Once a claim has been made, more information has to be provided elsewhere on the label. Some claims include the words "source of," "low in," "percent less," "light," "cholesterol free," and "low in saturated fat." But a food without cholesterol can still be very high in fat. A "light" food may have a light texture or taste rather than be light in fat.

3. The nutrition information provides nutrition details. These details refer to the product as it is sold and does not include other ingredients you may add at home. Since this labeling is voluntary, each product may provide different amounts of information. In the most complete labeling, you will find:
   - ☐ a. Serving size; tells you the amount of the food the nutrition information is based on. If you eat a larger serving than indicated, you will be eating more calories, salt, or other ingredients.
   - ☐ b. Energy tells you the calories (Kcal) per serving.
   - ☐ c. Fat indicates the total amount of fat in each serving. Some labels give the amount of the different types of fat: polyunsaturates, monounsaturates, saturates, cholesterol, and trans fats.
   - ☐ d. Carbohydrates may be listed alone or be broken down into sugars, starches, and fiber. If broken down, the sum of the parts will equal the total carbohydrate.

4. What about the grams? Information providing the grams of protein, carbohydrate, and fat in foods can be used to compare different food products. It can also be used to make decisions about purchasing a food based on the types of fat or carbohydrate that are in a food.

TAKING ACTION

Set realistic goals so you can be confident you will be able to keep this commitment to yourself. Review your responses to the Taking Stock quiz and think of small changes that will help you achieve a healthier lifestyle. Eating an extra piece of fruit a day instead of a dessert, weeding the garden, or walking to the shop are easy ways to introduce lifestyle improvements.

Set your own goals in the space below. It is your reminder of the action you've decided to take. Good luck!

My eating goals are:

1. _____

_____

2. _____

_____

3. _____

_____

WHAT YOU HAVE LEARNED IN THIS CHAPTER

- Weight loss is critical for dealing with metabolic syndrome.
- Focus on losing two pounds per week by eating 500 calories less per day and burning 500 calories with activity. Weight loss = more calories burned than calories consumed.
- Follow the optimal health food and energy pyramid for long-term, successful dietary changes.

In the next chapter we will learn how to incorporate physical activity into our day.

Chapter 11

FIT TO BE HEALTHY

A re you a couch potato? North Americans give new meaning to the term as more than sixty percent of the population do not participate in any form of regular physical activity, and twenty-five percent of all adults are not active at all. Physical inactivity goes hand in hand with obesity and is strongly linked to the development of metabolic syndrome. Physical inactivity is a serious nationwide problem. Researchers from the Centers for Disease Control and Prevention studied a total of 1,626 men and women aged twenty or older in the National Health and Nutrition Examination Survey. They found that those participants who did not engage in any moderate or vigorous physical activity during leisure time had almost twice the odds of having metabolic syndrome as those who reportedly engaged in more than 150 minutes per week of such activity.

We need to start making a conscious effort to increase physical activity, spend less time watching television, using computers, playing video games, and being overall lazy. Sedentary desk jobs have compounded the inactivity problem, as many of us sit at a desk all day, barely moving or leaving for lunch, because our coffee breaks involve e-mailing friends or talking on the phone. Our ancestors were physically active during the day, hunting for and gathering food. They didn't have modern-day transportation, which makes it easy for us to avoid activity. How many of us have driven around the parking lot at the grocery store until we found a spot closest to the door?

Physical activity helps your muscle cells use blood sugar, which they need for energy. Exercise makes those cells more sensitive to insulin, thereby preventing and controlling insulin resistance. A study in Finland found that men who exercised more than three hours per week decreased their risk of developing metabolic syndrome by about fifty percent compared with the men who exercised no more than sixty minutes per week. Regular physical activity has also been seen to reduce VLDL and LDL (bad) cholesterol, while raising HDL (good) cholesterol, lowering blood pressure, and reducing insulin resistance.

We all need to increase our physical activity levels, but this doesn't mean we should all become long-distance runners, join spin classes, or be the next heavy weight champion. The recommendation is fairly simple: thirty minutes of physical activity five times a week, which can result in weight loss, improved blood pressure, improved cholesterol levels, and a reduced risk of developing type 2 diabetes. An increase in physical activity causes a reduction in the risk factors for metabolic syndrome and independently reduces the risk of heart disease and improves cardiovascular fitness.

PHYSICAL ACTIVITY AND INSULIN RESISTANCE

Muscle is the most insulin-sensitive tissue in the body, and is therefore the main target for affecting insulin resistance. Physical training has been shown to reduce insulin resistance regardless of body mass index (BMI). The impact of exercise on insulin sensitivity is evident for twenty-four to forty-eight hours and disappears within three to five days. Thus, regular physical activity should be a part of any effort to reverse the effects of insulin resistance.

MELT AWAY FAT AND METABOLIC SYNDROME WITH EXERCISE

A study in 2005 at Johns Hopkins Medical Center showed that people 55 to 75 years of age can benefit from a moderate program of physical exercise. The reduced incidence of metabolic syndrome was linked to a decrease in total and abdominal body fat and an increase in muscle leanness.

The researchers studied a group of 104 older adults for six months. None of the participants had previous signs of cardiovascular disease. Half of the participants were randomly assigned to a control group that received a booklet on increased physical activity, such as walking, to promote good health. The other half participated in supervised exercise for sixty minutes three times per week. The combination of exercises was designed to work all major muscle groups and the heart, and to increase circulation. Exercises included aerobic activity on a treadmill, bicycle, or stair stepper, as well as weight lifting.

The researchers measured changes in body fat and in muscle and fitness levels. They found substantial improvements in the group that exercised for six months. The average weight loss in this group was four pounds, and much of the fat loss was offset by increased muscle mass. The fat in the stomach area was reduced by twenty percent. The waist is an important target area as abdominal fat is highly correlated to metabolic syndrome. People in the group that received the booklet and did not participate in supervised exercise had either no weight loss or significantly less improvement than those in the exercise group.

The researchers also saw a reduction of forty-one percent of metabolic syndrome cases in the exercising groups.

There is consensus that virtually all people can benefit from regular activity. Although physical activity and exercise are key factors in successful weight loss programs, the effects of exercise alone on weight loss are considerably less dramatic than those of caloric restriction alone. Still, exercise is a key determinant of successful long-term maintenance of weight loss.

EXERCISE LOWERS C-REACTIVE PROTEIN

In a study published in *Journal of the American College of Cardiology*, researchers assessed the physical fitness levels of 1,640 people and measured their C-reactive protein levels (protein produced by the liver, marker of inflammation, and associated with heart disease). About twenty percent of the participants had metabolic syndrome. The researchers found that those with metabolic syndrome who were physically fit had much lower C-reactive protein (CRP) levels than those who were inactive.

Among the most physically fit people with metabolic syndrome, the average CRP level was half as much as the average level among the least fit. In addition, the effect of physical fitness on CRP levels was more pronounced in people with metabolic syndrome than in healthy people.

This study shows that physical fitness has a positive influence on CRP levels, regardless of other risk factors. These findings and many others prove that those with metabolic syndrome need to increase their level of physical activity to reduce their risk of heart disease.

FITNESS LEVELS REDUCE RISK OF METABOLIC SYNDROME

High fitness levels provide sixty-three percent protection against metabolic syndrome even in individuals with increased susceptibility because of existing metabolic risk factors (for example, a BMI greater than 30, insulin resistance, high blood pressure, low HDL cholesterol, and high triglycerides). Cardiovascular fitness, as measured on a treadmill test, is a strong independent predictor of the risk of metabolic syndrome. The researchers of this study say that greater fitness could prevent people with some components of the metabolic syndrome from going on to develop the whole cluster of disorders. The findings are based on a study of 10, 498 subjects who had their cardiovascular fitness levels determined at baseline and were then followed for five years to assess the occurrence of metabolic syndrome.

In both sexes, the risk of metabolic syndrome fell as each successive fitness level was attained. For men, the middle and upper levels of fitness reduced the risk of metabolic syndrome by 26 and 53 percent respectively. The corresponding reductions in women were 20 and 63 percent.

In men, even those who had various metabolic syndrome components, increased fitness resulted in a significant improvement in metabolic syndrome risk. In women, the association was significant only if no components were present.

Getting Started

Physical activity is a critical component in preventing and or managing metabolic syndrome. We need to get off the couch and start moving. This does not mean you have to join a gym, spin class, or other structured program, but it does mean you need to incorporate at least thirty minutes of aerobic activity every day, or at a minimum five days a week. Recent evidence shows that the less structured the activity is, the more successful you will be in incorporating the recommended thirty minutes per day.

Increasing your physical activity will have dramatic benefits on your health in the following ways:

- decreases insulin resistance and can aid in preventing type 2 diabetes and cardiovascular disease; it can help you manage metabolic syndrome
- helps your body burn calories, which will help you lose weight
- decreases insulin resistance
- helps build and maintain healthy bones, muscles, and joints
- decreases body fat, especially abdominal fat (the fat that brings the greatest risk of developing metabolic syndrome)
- increases serotonin levels (serotonin is the feel-good, happy hormone)
- gives you a positive outlook on life
- improves sleep
- helps control stress levels

Those with type 2 diabetes or cardiovascular disease should undergo a clinical assessment and screening before beginning any exercise program, to ensure that they are in good enough condition to avoid injuries, especially if they have not engaged in physical activity until now. If you are older than thirty-five and have additional cardiovascular risk factors, vascular disease, long-standing disease, or neuropathy, you should have an exercise stress test. If you are on diabetes medications, you need to monitor blood sugar levels and adjust your diet to minimize fluctuations in blood sugar levels during exercise.

Tell Me How

The exercise program should consist of moderately intense aerobic exercises that can be sustained for thirty minutes or longer. Each exercise session should incorporate a five- to ten-minute warm-up and a five- to ten-minute post-exercise cooldown of low-intensity aerobic exercise (walking, cycling) or slow, rhythmic stretching exercises to prevent injuries. Depending on your level of physical conditioning, physical activity longer than thirty minutes as tolerated is encouraged.

For anyone who currently does no activity, starting even moderate, regular physical activity may be difficult. The daily physical activity target should be built up in small activity portions (ten to fifteen minutes) over time. The rate of progression will depend on several factors, including age, functional capacity, medical status, personal preferences, and goals. Begin with small increases in current activity and build up gradually. Remember, physical activity does not have to be strenuous to achieve health benefits.

TYPES OF ACTIVITIES

The preferred mode of aerobic exercise is brisk walking for a minimum of thirty minutes on most days of the week. As physical fitness improves and you become familiar with the sensations associated with aerobic training, other large-muscle activities, such as swimming, cycling, rowing, cross-country skiing, and aerobic dance, can be introduced to provide variety. Walking and some home-based activities, such as housework and gardening, are useful to increase strength, mobility, and cardiovascular fitness in the sedentary. They are ideal activities for most people as they require little or no equipment, expense, or skill, and are more likely to result in long-term behavioral changes. They can be incorporated into daily routines and can be started from a very low fitness base.

Non-weight-bearing activity may be appropriate for the obese (BMI of more than 30) to prevent injuries and protect joints. Stationary cycling, swimming, or aqua classes are all suitable. Fun, sociable, and regular activities that are not dependent on the season will increase commitment to healthy activity.

These and other activities—for example, stair climbing, hiking, calisthenics, bicycling, rowing, swimming, tennis, racquetball, soccer, basketball, and touch football—are especially beneficial when performed regularly.

WORK OUT SMART

Exercise is essential to help with weight loss and for overall health, but the age-old debate remains in terms of how much and what kind of exercise is best. Researchers at the University of Pittsburgh enrolled 201 overweight, sedentary women as participants in a one-year study. The women were assigned to one of four exercise groups: vigorous intensity with high duration; moderate intensity with high duration; moderate intensity with moderate duration; and vigorous intensity with moderate duration. All the women, regardless of which exercise group they were in ate 1,200 to 1,500 calories per day.

The researchers found that weight loss was significant in all groups. Those who exercised moderately gained benefits similar to those who exercised vigorously. Participants who walked briskly (moderate exercise) for at least fifty minutes, five times a week, and who cut back on fatty foods saw the best long-term weight loss. In six months, the women in this group lost an average of twenty-five pounds. So it isn't how hard you work, but how smart you work, that will help you get the greatest results.

Intensity: How Hard Do You Need to Work?

Effort should always be proportional to fitness: the simple rule of thumb is for an unconditioned individual to work at a comfortable level indicated by the continued ability to talk while breathing faster than normal and feeling warm.

The intensity should not produce adverse reactions during or after exercise. Many people dislike exercising because they overexert and feel uncomfortable or suffer injury. This is entirely unnecessary.

Table 11.1: Moderate-Level Physical Activities

Common Household Activities	Sport Activities
Washing and waxing a car for 45 to 60 minutes	Playing volleyball for 45-60 minutes
Gardening for 30 to 45 minutes	Walking 2 miles in 30 minutes
Raking leaves for 30 minutes	Social dancing (fast) for 30 minutes
Shoveling snow for 15 minutes	Water aerobics for 30 minutes
Stair walking for 15 minutes	Swimming laps for 20 minutes
Pushing a stroller 1.5 miles in 15 minutes	Jumping rope for 15 minutes
Washing floors for 45 minutes	Running 1.5 miles in 15 minutes

Sample Walking Program

Walking is one of the best and most recommended ways to incorporate physical activity into your day. The easiest way to get started is to start walking everywhere. I highly encourage people to buy a pedometer to track the number of steps they walk each day. The recommended goal is 10,000 steps per day. You would be amazed at how motivated to walk you will feel when you wear that pedometer—you want to continually see the number of steps climb on the meter. It is a very exciting feeling when you reach your daily goal.

You may also want to start a walking program to help keep you motivated and have a goal to work toward. Table 11.2 contains a sample program to help you build up muscle and endurance over time so you can reach the recommended thirty minutes or more. The plan includes a warm-up and cooldown, which are a must when doing any type of activity to prevent injury.

On the days you are not walking, I would recommend using light weights to incorporate some resistance training (building muscle helps you burn more calories and improve insulin sensitivity); and of course continue doing some of the common household chores that count toward meeting your goal of thirty minutes per day. Before long you will love how you feel after exercising. Exercise will become a regular part of your day, and you will find yourself missing it on the days you don't exercise.

Table 11.2: Sample Walking Program

	Warm-up	Activity	Cooldown	Total Time
WEEK 1				
Session A	Walk slowly 5 min.	Then walk briskly 5 min.	Then walk slowly 5 min.	15 min.
Session B	Repeat above pattern			
Session C	Repeat above pattern			
Continue with at least three walking sessions during each week of the program.				
WEEK 2	Walk slowly 5 min.	Then walk briskly 7 min.	Then walk slowly 5 min.	17 min.
WEEK 3	Walk slowly 5 min.	Then walk briskly 9 min.	Then walk slowly 5 min.	19 min.
WEEK 4	Walk slowly 5 min.	Then walk briskly 11 min.	Then walk slowly 5 min.	21 min.
WEEK 5	Walk slowly 5 min.	Then walk briskly 13 min.	Then walk slowly 5 min.	23 min.
WEEK 6	Walk slowly 5 min.	Then walk briskly 15 min.	Then walk slowly 5 min.	25 min.
WEEK 7	Walk slowly 5 min.	Then walk briskly 18 min.	Then walk slowly 5 min.	28 min.
WEEK 8	Walk slowly 5 min.	Then walk briskly 20 min.	Then walk slowly 5 min.	30 min.
WEEK 9	Walk slowly 5 min.	Then walk briskly 23 min.	Then walk slowly 5 min.	33 min.
WEEK 10	Walk slowly 5 min.	Then walk briskly 26 min.	Then walk slowly 5 min.	36 min.
WEEK 11	Walk slowly 5 min.	Then walk briskly 28 min.	Then walk slowly 5 min.	38 min.
WEEK 12 AND BEYOND	Walk slowly 5 min.	Then walk briskly 30 min.	Then walk slowly 5 min.	40 min.

What's a Pedometer?
A pedometer senses your body's motion and counts your footsteps. This count can be converted into distance if you measure the length of your usual stride. Wearing a pedometer and recording your daily steps and distance are great motivating tools. You can wear a pedometer all day, every day, and record total steps. Or you can wear it just when you go out for a walking workout.

For long-term health and reduced chronic disease—10,000 steps a day
For successful, sustained weight loss—12,000 to 15,000 steps a day
To build aerobic fitness—3,000 or more fast steps a day

Be Physically Active
Place a checkmark next to the ways you will incorporate activity into your day.

❑ I'll take the stairs instead of the elevator.
❑ I'll find an activity I enjoy, for example walking, dancing, or swimming.
❑ I'll be active around the house—I'll wash the floors by hand or work in the garden.
❑ I'll walk the dog several days per week.
❑ I'll park at the far end of the shopping center lot and walk to the store.
❑ I'll take a walk every day, accumulating up to 30 minutes per day at least 5 days per week.
❑ I'll try strength training by lifting light weights 3 times per week.
❑ I'll wear a pedometer and reach the goal of 10,000 steps per day.
❑ I'll join a gym.
❑ I'll use one of my coffee breaks at work to do some type of aerobic activity.
❑ I'll start encouraging my friends to get active with me. Having another person to motivate me will go a long way.

WHAT YOU HAVE LEARNED IN THIS CHAPTER

- More than sixty percent of adults are not regularly physically active; twenty-five percent of adults are not active at all.

- Significant health benefits can be obtained by including a moderate amount of physical activity (for example, 30 minutes of brisk walking or raking leaves, 15 minutes of running, or 45 minutes of playing volleyball) on most, if not all, days of the week.

- Regular physical activity can prevent and or manage metabolic syndrome, type 2 diabetes, and cardiovascular disease.

Chapter 12

THE POWER OF
NATURAL SUPPLEMENTS

"Let food be thy medicine and thy medicine be thy food," said Hippocrates, the father of modern medicine 2,500 years ago. However, with the current state of the standard diet, and the available food supply providing a plethora of junk food and refined and processed foods, it is difficult to have traditional food be the medicine we need it to be. Natural supplements (nutrients that are normally found in food that are extracted into supplement form) can help prevent and treat many of today's modern diseases.

Combining healthy food choices, (see Chapter 10), with supplements is the best plan. In today's society it is difficult to rely on just one or the other; it's the combination that will help prevent disease. And it isn't just one particular supplement that will do the trick; depending on your dietary deficiencies, multiple nutrients may be required. Science has shown that excess insulin causes your body to become deficient in many vitamins, minerals, and other nutrients.

For those with metabolic syndrome, there are numerous research studies examining the power of natural supplements to help control insulin resistance and the complications that may arise, mainly diabetes and cardiovascular disease. It has been proven that a deficiency of many nutrients, which will be discussed in this chapter, are directly linked to insulin resistance and the development of metabolic syndrome.

Before you begin any supplement program for metabolic syndrome, diabetes, or weight loss, be sure to check with your physician, pharmacist, or naturopathic doctor. If you are pregnant, do not use any herbal supplements before checking with your doctor.

INSULIN RESPONSE

To prevent and treat metabolic syndrome, it is essential to improve insulin sensitivity. Numerous vitamins, minerals, and herbs have been studied to discover their influence on your body's response to insulin, thereby improving insulin sensitivity.

Chromium Picolinate

Chromium is an essential trace mineral required by the human body for normal carbohydrate and fat metabolism and without a doubt the most important mineral in the prevention and treatment of insulin resistance and metabolic syndrome. According to analysis of data from the United States Department of Agriculture (USDA), the average North American diet is low in chromium. This isn't surprising, since nutritional chromium is found in very low quantities in foods, and even this low amount can be compromised by modern processing and cooking methods. Another factor for chromium deficiencies is rising sugar consumption, which reduces chromium reserves in the body. There is a reduced level of nutritional chromium in foods because of the chromium-depleted soils in which our food is grown. Exacerbating the situation is the fact that absorption of chromium from the diet is poor: less than 2.5 percent of ingested chromium is absorbed. Aging is associated with a 25 to 40 percent drop in chromium levels. Chromium deficiency may be implicated in age-onset type 2 diabetes.

Chromium picolinate is the most popular form of supplemental chromium. Picolinate, a by-product of the amino acid tryptophan, is paired with chromium in supplements because the picolinate may help the body absorb chromium more efficiently. Chromium is important in the breakdown of carbohydrates and fats, and it helps cells respond properly to insulin. High levels of circulating insulin, as seen in those with insulin resistance and metabolic syndrome, may deplete the body's chromium stores.

Some research has shown that without chromium, insulin's actions may be blocked and glucose levels may become elevated. The surface of the body's cells become resistant to insulin and require chromium to function properly. Chromium supplements have been shown to effectively maintain insulin function by activating insulin receptor cells. Chromium helps insulin open the door to the cell membrane, thus allowing glucose to enter the cells.

More than twenty clinical studies of more than 2,000 diabetic subjects support the ability of chromium to improve blood glucose (glycemic control), enhance insulin sensitivity, and improve lipid (triglycerides, cholesterol levels) in people with diabetes.

A new, preclinical study, conducted at the University of Alberta and presented at the third World Congress on Insulin Resistance Syndrome, is the first of its kind to show that chromium picolinate may improve the overall health of the circulatory system in those with prediabetes or insulin resistance. The animal study showed that daily treatment with chromium picolinate increased relaxation of the blood vessels and improved blood flow to the heart. This is very encouraging as those with prediabetes and insulin resistance have 1.5 times as much risk of cardiovascular disease as those people with normal blood sugar levels. Taking chromium picolinate daily may alter that state and prevent cardiovascular disease from developing.

Recommended dose: 200 to 1,000 mcg per day. See supplement chart for further information.

Biotin

Biotin is a water-soluble member of the B-complex group of vitamins and is necessary for both metabolism and growth in humans, particularly in the production of fats, antibodies, and digestive enzymes. In people with diabetes, biotin can help regulate insulin levels; it improves beta cell function (the cells of the pancreas responsible for releasing insulin).

Recommended dose: 9 mg per day.

Combination of Chromium and Biotin

New research indicates that the combination of chromium picolinate and biotin may improve cardiovascular risk factors and support glycemic control. The combination shows enhanced ability to combat insulin resistance risk factors and enhance glucose uptake in people with type 2 diabetes.

A 30-day rapid response to this combination has been demonstrated in controlled studies measuring fasting blood sugar and coronary risk factors. A 454-patient, double-blind, placebo-controlled study was conducted by the nation's fifth largest diabetes disease-management company. The results showed that subjects taking chromium picolinate plus biotin had notable improvements in HbA1c (measurement of long-term blood-sugar levels should be lower than seven percent), total cholesterol, and in the triglycerides/high-density lipoprotein ratio compared to those taking the placebo.

Chromium and biotin act synergistically to improve insulin sensitivity and glucose tolerance.

Recommended combination: 600 mcg chromium picolinate plus 2 mg biotin per day.

Zinc

Zinc deficiency is rare in developed countries; however, many people in North America may be at risk for a zinc deficiency. Zinc plays an important role in glucose regulation; the proper function of insulin (it helps the pancreas produce insulin and allows insulin to work more efficiently); and weight control.

Studies have reported that low zinc intake is associated with several of the risk factors common in metabolic syndrome, and a low blood level of zinc is associated with insulin resistance in overweight people. Research has shown that zinc may positively affect blood levels of leptin. Leptin is a hormone that influences appetite and energy expenditure. Zinc also provides antioxidant protection and is an important agent in wound healing and the prevention of infections.

Recommended dose: 30 to 60 mg zinc per day.

Magnesium

Like chromium, magnesium is involved in glucose metabolism and in the prevention of metabolic syndrome. Magnesium is necessary for the production and release of insulin and is also required by the cells for maintaining insulin sensitivity and increasing the number of insulin receptors. Magnesium deficiency can reduce insulin sensitivity, and low dietary intake and low blood levels of magnesium have been associated with greater insulin resistance in non-diabetic people.

As important as magnesium is, at least half of North Americans do not consume the recommended level of magnesium, and the low levels of magnesium in our diet increase the risk of developing insulin resistance and metabolic syndrome. Most of the magnesium we need should be derived from our diet; it is abundant in whole foods (tofu, legumes, seeds, nuts, whole grains, and green leafy vegetables), but lacking in refined, processed foods.

Recommended dose: 300 to 500 mg per day in the form of magnesium aspartate or citrate and a magnesium-rich diet.

Vanadyl Sulphate

Studies in animals who do not have diabetes suggest that vanadium may have an insulin-like effect, reducing blood sugar levels and increasing cellular insulin sensitivity. Based on these findings, preliminary studies involving humans have been conducted with promising results. Doctors at Toronto's Mount Sinai Hospital found that vanadyl sulphate promotes insulin action by three mechanisms: directly mimicking insulin action, enhancing insulin sensitivity, and prolonging insulin's biological response.

In Japan, researchers reported success with animal studies involving diabetic rats and vanadyl sulphate. When administered in high doses, vanadyl sulphate was shown to decrease blood glucose levels by 67 percent within two days. Levels remained low for at least 12 weeks without affecting low plasma insulin levels.

Recommended dose: 25 to 50 mg per day.

Cinnamon

Cinnamon may significantly help people with type 2 diabetes improve their ability to respond to insulin, thus normalizing their blood sugar levels. Data from the Agricultural Research Unit in Maryland was first published in the *New Scientist* in August 2000. The researchers found that, in diabetics, cinnamon rekindled the ability of fat cells to respond to insulin and greatly increased glucose removal. It is believed that a substance in cinnamon called MHCP is the main reason for its beneficial results. Both test-tube and animal studies have shown that compounds in cinnamon not only stimulate insulin receptors, but also inhibit an enzyme that inactivates them, thus significantly increasing the ability to use glucose. A study of thirty people with type 2 diabetes revealed a significant decrease in blood glucose, triglycerides, LDL, and cholesterol levels after the people took cinnamon for forty days. These studies have shown that less than half a teaspoon per day of cinnamon reduces blood sugar levels in persons with type 2 diabetes.

Recommended dose: 1/2 tsp per day. Cinnamon is also available in supplemental form.

Gymnema Sylvestre

Gymnema is a traditional Ayurvedic herb with a 3,000-year history of balancing elevated blood sugar levels. This woody, vinelike plant is known in India as the "destroyer of sugar." The active ingredients, gymnemic acid and gurmarin, have molecular structures similar to glucose and are beneficial in many ways. Gurmarin has the ability to fill taste bud receptors and reduce the sweet taste of sugary foods, which greatly reduces the craving for sweets. Gymnemic acid helps increase the production of insulin by stimulating the production of new insulin-promoting beta cells in the pancreas. Gymnemic acid also facilitates insulin release from the beta cells into the bloodstream by increasing beta-cell membrane permeability. Gymnemic acid also inhibits the absorption of sugar molecules in the intestines during digestion, thus reducing increases in blood sugar levels.

Recommended dose: 400 mg per day.

Bitter Melon (Momordica Charantin)

Bitter melon, also called bitter gourd, bitter cucumber, balsam pear, karela, and charantin, has been used in many cultures for centuries to treat diabetes. Momordica contains insulin-like polypeptide, which lowers the blood glucose. The effects of Momordica on fasting and postprandial (after eating) blood glucose levels were studied in 100 people with type 2 diabetes. Consuming bitter melon in juice form led to significant reduction of both fasting and postprandial serum glucose levels. This hypoglycemic action was observed in 86 percent of cases; 5 percent showed lowering of fasting serum glucose only.

The hypoglycemic influence of Momordica is claimed to be mediated through an insulin secretory effect or through an influence on enzymes involved in glucose metabolism. It is believed that bitter melon acts on the pancreatic cells and the non-pancreatic cells like muscles.

Fresh bitter melon is available at many Asian grocery stores. Look for a melon that is pale green or yellow (orange melons are too old). Slice the unpeeled fruit lengthwise, remove the seeds, cut the melon into thin slices, and steam or boil them until the fruit is tender enough to cut with the edge of a spoon. Place the fruit with an equal amount of water in a blender and puree for two minutes. Drink. Or substitute bitter melon juice, found in Asian grocery stores.

Recommended dose: Prepared melon, 1/4 to 1/2 cup per day Liquid extract,1/4 to 1/2 tsp up to three times daily. You can also utilize bitter melon supplements standardized to 2.5% bitters including charantins. Aim for 3 x 500 mg capsules per day.

Fenugreek

The seeds of fenugreek are a condiment commonly used in Indian homes and are a rich source of fiber, particularly the gel fiber known as mucilage, which is thought to be responsible for the hypoglycemic effect. Fenugreek is part of the legume family, which includes chickpeas, peanuts, and green peas. It is thought to delay gastric emptying, to slow carbohydrate absorption, and to inhibit glucose transport. Fenugreek seeds exert blood sugar-lowering effects by stimulating insulin secretion from pancreatic cells.

In a study of sixty people with type 2 diabetes, 25 grams per day of fenugreek led to significant improvements in overall blood sugar control, and lowered blood sugar elevations in response to a meal. It also lowered cholesterol levels.

In another two-month study of twenty-five individuals with type 2 diabetes, use of fenugreek (1 gram of standardized extract) significantly improved some measures of blood sugar control and insulin response compared to placebo. Triglyceride levels decreased and HDL (good) cholesterol levels increased, presumably due to the enhanced insulin sensitivity.

Recommended dose: 5 to 30 grams of defatted fenugreek seeds three times per day with meals, or 1 gram of fenugreek extract per day.

Vitamin B6

Vitamin B6, also called pyridoxine, helps the body convert carbohydrates into sugar, which is burned to produce energy. B vitamins are essential in the metabolism of fats and protein.

Many diabetics have low levels of vitamin B6, and levels are even lower in those with diabetic neuropathy. In a study of people with diabetes, those who received pyridoxine alpha-ketoglutarate (a form of vitamin B6) for one month experienced significant reductions in fasting blood sugar levels compared to those who did not receive the supplement.

Shortages of the B vitamins can also lead to nerve damage in the hands and feet. Some studies indicate that people with diabetes experience less of the numbness and tingling of diabetes-caused nerve damage if they get supplemental amounts of B vitamins such as B6 and B12.

Recommended dose: 1.8 grams per day.

Ginseng

The term ginseng refers to several species of the genus *Panax*. For more than two thousand years, the roots of this slow-growing plant have been valued in Chinese medicine. The two most commonly used species are Korean ginseng (*Panax ginseng*) and American ginseng (*Panax quinquefolius*). American ginseng decreases fatigue and aids in the feeling of well-being and is prescribed for a variety of problems including stress, failing memory, obesity, flagging vitality, exhaustion, improving the immune system, fatigue, and improving fertility and virility. Ginseng is also used as a general strengthening tonic for the body.

Studies have shown American ginseng helps increase energy and normalize blood sugar levels if three grams are taken before each meal.

Korean ginseng lowers blood sugar levels in diabetics by improving insulin sensitivity, a known problem for those with type 2 diabetics. Korean ginseng is a natural stimulant; it increases energy and helps people lose weight.

Recommended dose: American ginseng, 3 grams before each meal. Korean ginseng, 200 mg per day of the standardized extract or 0.5 to 2 g per day of the dry root. Only recommended for type 2 diabetes and not type 1.

GLYCEMIC RESPONSE

The glycemic response of a food or nutrient is based on its ability to raise blood sugar levels. Depending on what type of carbohydrate it is, it will affect how quickly blood sugar is raised. This blood sugar-raising effect of food is indicated by the glycemic index (for more information see the Appendix). Aim for foods that provide a slower rise in blood glucose, such as legumes, nuts, and whole-grain carbohydrates, as opposed to simple and refined sugars like white bread.

Viscofiber

Viscofiber is a high-beta-glucan concentrate derived from either barley or oats that have uncharacteristic high viscosity. The importance of viscosity has been accepted by the FDA and well documented by leading fiber scientists as the major property responsible for the physiological effects of consuming viscous soluble fiber.

The mechanism of how beta glucan works in the body is well understood and attributed to viscous soluble fiber, followed by insoluble fibers and accompanying substances. Viscofiber has all these unique characteristics, resulting in multiple heart health benefits.

The high viscosity of Viscofiber increases the duration of intestinal transit and delays digestion of available carbohydrates, leading to a reduction of glycemic response. Multiple clinical trials using Viscofiber have demonstrated a dose response effect for improving glucose and insulin levels. Viscofiber oat is 50 percent beta glucan, and Viscofiber barley is 60 percent beta glucan. The more beta glucan consumed, the better the results. Viscofiber is viscoussoluble fiber, so ensure adequate fluids are taken.

Recommended dose: 2 grams of beta glucan per day.

NEUROPATHY

Neuropathy is nerve damage caused by prolonged high blood sugar levels. It results in numbness and pain in the extremities, but it can also affect internal organs, such as the digestive tract, heart, and sexual organs. Diabetes is the leading cause of erectile dysfunction in men.

Close regulation of blood sugar is the best way to prevent neuropathy. There is no cure, but researchers have said that borage oil is one of the best ways to prevent and treat it.

Borage Oil

Borage oil contains the important omega-6 fatty acid gamma linolenic acid, or GLA, which has been shown to be one of the best natural remedies available for the prevention and treatment of diabetic neuropathy. Four to fifty percent of diabetics will have to cope with neuropathy, which is the leading cause of amputations in the United States.

The body utilizes GLA to build a healthy nerve structure. Diabetics have a difficult time metabolizing the omega-6 linoleic acid, which we receive from our diet, into the important GLA. The result is a lower level of GLA.

Human clinical studies have concluded that GLA has a beneficial effect on the course of diabetic neuropathy. Trials began in 1986, when a group of researchers conducted a double-blind, placebo-controlled study with twenty-two patients. The treatment group received 360 mg of GLA per day for six months. All tested variables, including peripheral nerve function, nerve conduction speed, and nerve capillary blood flow, improved in the treatment group and worsened in the control group.

Two subsequent multicenter studies, involving more than 400 patients, obtained consistently positive results. The first included 11 patients in seven centers, while the second included 293 patients in ten centers. The patients received 480 mg of GLA daily for one year. The researchers measured sixteen variables in all, including nerve conduction strength and speed, hot and cold thresholds, sensation, reflexes, and muscle strength. After a full year of treatment, all sixteen variables showed favorable improvement compared to the control group.

Research indicates that recovery of patients may be even more complete when GLA is used in conjunction with antioxidants. An animal study combining GLA with alpha lipoic acid showed that subjects had great improvement in the motor skills and blood flow deficits associated with neuropathy. Researchers noted that this synergistic combination far outweighed the effects of either supplement used separately.

GLA has also been shown to help people lose weight—an important factor when preventing diabetes and heart disease. GLA activates a metabolic process that can burn close to half of the body's total calories. In one GLA study, individuals lost from 9.6 to 11.4 pounds over a six-week period.

Not only does GLA help with weight loss, it also improves lipid profiles and other risk factors for cardiovascular disease, such as blood pressure.

Recommended dose: 500 mg GLA per day (found in 2 to 3 g borage capsules) for neuropathy and treating insulin resistance. For the prevention of insulin resistance, consume 240 mg GLA daily (1 g borage). For weight loss, heart disease, and metabolic syndrome, 1 g GLA (4 g borage oil daily) or 8 g evening primrose oil.

LIPID LEVELS

Abnormal cholesterol and triglyceride levels are components of the metabolic syndrome and cardiovascular disease. Many diabetics also suffer from abnormal lipid levels. Dietary changes and many nutrients can help keep your cholesterol and triglycerides in check, one of the best ones being the omega-3 fatty acids from fish.

Omega-3s

Omega-3s may benefit people with diabetes by improving glucose tolerance levels and providing cardioprotective effects, including reduced cardiovascular mortality, by improving circulation, platelet aggregation, and triglyceride reduction. Omega-3s benefit the entire body by creating fluid cell membranes, which help increase blood flow, improve nutrient and vitamin absorption, and prevent and treat numerous types of diseases, including rheumatoid arthritis, depression, asthma, attention deficit disorder, psoriasis, and some cancers. To delay and prevent disease, it is critical to have a cell structure composed of unsaturated fats instead of saturated or trans fats.

Omega-3s in the form of high-quality, toxin-free fish oil provide the highest level of long-chain polyunsaturated fatty acids available. Large clinical and population-based studies have been conducted on the benefits of omega-3s for people with cardiovascular disease and diabetes. Results are conclusive: fish oil offers protection against heart disease in people with diabetes and those without. My preference is fish oil over flax oil as a source of omega-3s, especially for diabetes and cardiovascular disease prevention and treatment.

It is important to increase your weekly consumption of high-quality fatty fish, for example wild salmon or tuna. However, adding a fish oil supplement to your daily regime ensures that you are getting sufficient levels of these important fatty acids. The American Heart Association endorses the use of fish oil supplements for the prevention of heart disease and for the treatment of high triglyceride levels.

Recommended dose: 1 gram omega-3s (Eicosapentaenoic acid, EPA, and docosahexaenoic acid, DHA) per day for the prevention and treatment of insulin resistance, metabolic syndrome, and cardiovascular disease. To lower triglyceride levels, increase dose to 2 to 3 g per day of total omega-3s. Look for fish oils utilizing sardine, anchovy, and mackerel combinations in at least a 50% total omega-3 concentration. Therefore, a 1 g capsule would provide 500 mg of omega-3s, and you would take 2 capsules per day. The higher the concentration of omega-3s, the better.

Viscofiber

Upon being consumed, the oat-and-barley soluble fiber called Viscofiber forms a gel in the small intestine that surrounds bile acids and prevents them from being reabsorbed through the walls of the small intestine and recycled to the liver. The bile acids are trapped by the gel and excreted from the body, forcing the liver to take cholesterol out of the blood to replace the bile acids that have been excreted. The result is reduced total and LDL cholesterol.

Recommended dose: FDA recommended dose is 3 g beta glucan 0.75 g per dose. However, the more beta glucan consumed, the greater the results.

Fenugreek

Fenugreek contains soluble fiber—called mucilage—thought to lower total cholesterol and raise HDL cholesterol levels in diabetic individuals. Researchers at the S.N. Medical College in Agra, India, measured cholesterol levels of sixty type 2 (non-insulin-dependent) diabetics who were not taking any diabetes or cholesterol-lowering medication. Participants were asked to eat a bowl of soup containing about one ounce of powdered fenugreek seed before their lunch and dinner. After four weeks of consuming about two ounces of powdered fenugreek seed soup daily, the participants' cholesterol levels began to decline. After twenty-four weeks, their average total cholesterol was down fourteen percent, LDLs declined fifteen percent, and HDLs rose ten percent. Those with the highest cholesterol levels initially showed even greater benefit.

Recommended dose: 5 to 30 g defatted fenugreek seeds 3 times per day with meals, or 1 g fenugreek standardized extract.

Niacin

Niacin, also known as vitamin B3, has been shown to lower LDL cholesterol and triglycerides while raising HDL cholesterol. All B vitamins help the body convert carbohydrates into blood sugar, which is then burned to produce energy. They are also essential in the breakdown of protein and fats. Niacin is also used to prevent the development of plaque on the blood vessel walls (atherosclerosis), and to prevent any further blood vessel damage. According to a review of major clinical trials, the use of niacin for the prevention and treatment of atherosclerosis is based on strong and consistent science.

Niacin is so effective for cholesterol reduction that it has been compared side by side to popular cholesterol-lowering drugs and has shown a greater overall effect. In a study published in *The New England Journal of Medicine*, when simvastatin (Zocor) and niacin are combined, heart disease can be slowed and in some cases reversed. Although I don't recommend cholesterol-lowering drugs, sometimes they are necessary, especially initially and if cholesterol levels are higher than 240 mg/dl.

Because diabetes is often associated with atherosclerosis and abnormal cholesterol levels, all three conditions can benefit from nutrients that help manage cholesterol levels. There has been some concern, based on recent clinical research, that large doses of niacin (3 g) may increase blood sugar levels, but hemoglobin A1C (the blood protein that is an accurate marker of long-term blood sugar levels) decreased. If you are a diabetic, make sure you consult your health care provider before starting large doses of niacin.

Many people have difficulty tolerating niacin because of the skin-flushing effect. This can be avoided by taking niacin just before going to bed; most people will sleep through the reaction. You may also want to try the time-released forms of niacin, which may help minimize any potential reactions.

Recommended dose: 1.5 to 3 g per day, divided throughout the day.

Vitamin B6

Low dietary intake of vitamin B6 is associated with higher risk of heart disease. This may be because vitamin B6, vitamin B9 (folic acid), and vitamin B12 together help keep homocysteine levels under control. Homocysteine is an amino acid. Elevated levels of this amino acid are associated with increased risk of heart disease and stroke.

The American Heart Association recommends that most people obtain enough of these important B vitamins from the diet (bananas, avocadoes, brewer's yeast, chicken, pork, fish, and beef), rather than taking supplements. Under certain circumstances, however, supplements may be necessary. Such circumstances include elevated homocysteine levels with known heart disease or strong family history of heart disease at a young age.

Recommended dose: 50 mg per day.

Garlic

Garlic (*allium sativum*) possesses powerful medicinal properties (the active compound is called allicin). Garlic has an effect on cholesterol and triglyceride levels. Onions contain some of the same active ingredients, but in much lower doses. Modern medical science suggests one reason garlic might reduce cholesterol is that garlic is a proven antioxidant. This property might help prevent LDLs from being oxidized. In this way the cholesterol buildup that clogs the arteries could perhaps be reduced by garlic.

Studies have found garlic to lower cholesterol by an average of 9 to 12 percent; however, the results are not always consistent. This could be in part because of the different quality and type of garlic used. Garlic also functions as a natural blood thinner by reducing the body's production of thromboxane compounds, which stimulate blood clotting.

Recommended dose: 5,000 mcg allicin per day.

Polymethoxylated Flavones

Polymethoxylated flavones, naturally derived from citrus and palm fruits, have been shown in clinical studies to deliver impressive cardiovascular benefits because of their ability to positively affect the amount of cholesterol and triglycerides produced by the body. Overproduction of cholesterol is one of the reasons many people have trouble maintaining healthy levels through diet and exercise alone.

Recommended dose: 300 mg polymethoxylated flavones per day.

ANTIOXIDANTS

Vitamin E

Vitamin E is a fat-soluble vitamin present in many foods, especially green leafy vegetables, nuts, fats, and oils. It is one of a number of nutrients called antioxidants. Some other well-known antioxidants include vitamin C and beta-carotene. Antioxidants are nutrients that block some of the damage caused by toxic by-products released when the body transforms food into energy or fights off infection. The buildup of these by-products over time is largely responsible for the aging process and can contribute to the development of various health conditions such as heart disease, cancer, and a host of inflammatory conditions such as arthritis. Vitamin E can reduce oxidation, which makes LDL cholesterol more likely to collect and form plaque inside artery walls.

People who eat a diet rich in vitamin E are less likely to develop diabetes. Vitamin E has been shown to increase insulin sensitivity in both healthy people and in those with high blood pressure. Antioxidants, especially vitamin E, have been found to inhibit LDL cholesterol.

In a study published in *Diabetes Care* researchers followed 2,285 men and 2,019 women for more than twenty years. At the beginning of the study, all the participants were between 40 and 69 years old, and none had diabetes. During a twenty-three-year follow-up, 164 men and 219 women developed type 2 diabetes. This is the most common type of diabetes and is most commonly found in people older than forty who are overweight and do not get enough exercise.

The study found that vitamin E intake was significantly associated with a reduced risk of type 2 diabetes. In fact those who included the largest amounts of vitamin E in their diets were thirty percent less likely to develop the condition, compared to those who included the least amount.

Another study published in *Diabetes Care* indicated that about forty percent of diabetic patients can reduce their risk of heart attacks and of dying from heart disease by taking vitamin E supplements.

Make sure you take the natural form of vitamin E, which is called d-alpha-tocopherol.

Recommended dose: 800 to 1350 mg per day.

Vitamin C

Vitamin C is a water-soluble vitamin needed for the growth and repair of tissues in all parts of the body. It is necessary to form collagen, an important protein used to make skin, scar tissue, tendons, ligaments, and blood vessels. Vitamin C is essential for the healing of wounds and for the repair and maintenance of cartilage, bones, and teeth.

The body does not manufacture vitamin C on its own, nor does it store it. It is therefore important to include plenty of vitamin C-containing foods in your daily diet. Fresh fruits and vegetables are the best sources. Large amounts of vitamin C are used by the body during any kind of healing process, whether it's from an infection, disease, injury, or surgery.

Vitamin C may help people with diabetes in a number of ways. Some studies suggest that people with diabetes have high levels of free radicals and low levels of antioxidants, including vitamin C. This imbalance may partly explain why people with diabetes are at greater risk for developing conditions such as high cholesterol and atherosclerosis.

Insulin helps cells in the body take up the vitamin C the cells need to function properly. At the same time, lots of circulating blood sugar, as is often present in diabetics, prevents the cells from getting the vitamin C they need, even if the person is eating lots of fruits and vegetables. For this reason, taking extra vitamin C in the form of supplements may help those with diabetes.

People who eat foods rich in antioxidants, including vitamin C, are less prone to high blood pressure than people without these nutritious foods in their diet. Vitamin C may help protect blood vessels from the damaging effects that lead to or result from the presence of atherosclerosis. People with low levels of vitamin C may be more likely to have a heart attack or stroke.

Recommended dose: 500 to 1000 mg per day.

Coenzyme Q10 (CoQ10)

Although best known for its cardiovascular benefits, CoQ10 is essential in creating the spark that ignites fatty acid oxidation (fat burning). CoQ10 also acts as a powerful antioxidant inside the mitochondria (where the majority of free radicals are formed).

A double-blind trial showed that 120 mg CoQ10 per day reduced glucose and insulin blood levels in people with high blood pressure and heart disease. These results suggest that CoQ10 may improve insulin sensitivity in people with components of metabolic syndrome.

Recommended dose: 60 to 120 mg per day.

ALPHA LIPOIC ACID (ALA)

ALA, one of the most powerful and versatile antioxidants, also helps increase overall ATP (Adenosine triphosphate–cellular energy) levels, thus enhancing energy levels. Research from the Linus Pauling Institute, published in *Proceedings of the National Academy of Sciences* (2002), indicates that ALA in association with L-carnitine can greatly increase energy production and reverse the negative energy decline associated with aging.

Recommended dose: 50 to 300 mg daily.

WEIGHT LOSS

Losing weight and improving metabolic syndrome will yield many benefits, including higher HDL, lower triglycerides, less inflammation, improved insulin sensitivity, and lower blood pressure. The amount of weight loss required to improve metabolic syndrome and decrease blood pressure varies among individuals. Some people experience dramatic improvement in all measures with a modest loss of ten pounds, while others may need to lose significantly more weight to achieve the desired effects.

The Natural Medicines Comprehensive Database indicates that more than 50 individual dietary supplements and more than 125 commercial combination products are commonly used for weight loss. Some of the more commonly used supplements for weight loss have mild to moderate results. They are classified according to their proposed mechanism of action for weight loss. However, you should not look at these nutrients as the next "magic bullet" for weight loss, then forget about everything else you have read or learned throughout this book on lifestyle and diet changes. These nutrients are merely adjuncts to a healthy diet and exercise program; one can't replace the other. The bottom line is you must make dietary changes, and you must exercise. If you burn more calories than you eat, you will lose weight. There is no such thing as an easy way out when it comes to weight loss.

Increasing Satiety

Nutrients that are designed to increase satiety work by expanding in your gut where they absorb water and create a feeling of fullness, resulting in a lower calorie intake. Many fibrous products provide these results. However, glucomannan delivers the most impressive results.

Glucomannan

This unique soluble fiber comes from konjac root. It soaks up huge quantities of water. When taken as a capsule, it provides the effect of filling the stomach and creating a feeling of fullness and satiety. The result: your appetite is diminished, and you eat less. Glucomannan works best when taken with plenty of water before meals. People using glucomannan alone and without a specific diet program generally lose four to seven pounds a month.

In an eight-week, double-blind study, twenty obese subjects received one gram of glucomannan or a placebo daily. Subjects were instructed to not change eating or exercise habits. Glucomannan-supplemented subjects had a significant mean weight loss of 5.5 pounds. Total and LDL cholesterol were significantly reduced in the treated group.

In a three-month study of severely obese patients, a low-calorie diet by itself was tested against the same low-calorie diet in combination with three grams of glucomannan (in three doses) daily. The combination therapy resulted in more significant weight loss in relation to fatty mass alone, in an overall improvement in lipid status and carbohydrate tolerance, and in a greater adherence to the diet. The researchers concluded that "due to the marked ability to satiate patients and the positive metabolic effects, glucomannan diet supplements have been found to be particularly efficacious and well tolerated even in the long-term treatment of severe obesity."

Glucomannan has also been shown to reduce many of the risk factors in people with metabolic syndrome. One study found that 8 to 13 grams per day of glucomannan significantly improved several measures of blood cholesterol control and one measure of blood glucose control in people with metabolic syndrome.

Recommend dose: 1 g 3 times daily. Glucomannan must be taken with adequate amounts of fluids. Inadequate fluid may cause glucomannan to swell and block the throat, esophagus, or intestines.

Protein

Protein can reduce hunger (thereby decreasing the calories you consume), help you preserve muscle as you lose weight, and help your body build more muscle, particularly if you include strength training. A six-month study published in the *International Journal of Obesity* in 1999 compared two low-calorie diets: one with 12 percent of calories from protein and one with 25 percent of calories from protein. Those who ate more protein lost more weight. The subjects did not exercise.

You'll see weight-loss benefits by consuming either protein-rich foods or shakes, but shakes contain fewer calories and less fat than some high-protein foods, and they're also convenient.

Recommended dose: 20 to 25 g whey protein 2 to 3 times daily, preferably between meals. Drink one shake mid-morning and another an hour before dinner, which will help control your appetite at common craving times. Ensure that each meal contains a protein-rich food.

Increasing Energy Expenditure

Certain nutrients can help increase your metabolism and the number of calories burned in the day. This is an effective way to achieve weight loss.

Guarana

Guarana is made from the seeds of a plant native to Brazil. Guarana speeds up the brain's activity and is used to promote weight loss because of its stimulant and diuretic effect. It may also have some effect on increasing metabolism, suppressing appetite, and enhancing both mental and physical performance. Guarana contains 2.5 to 5 percent caffeine.

Most of the scientific evidence on caffeine as a general stimulant and an aid to exercise performance shows convincingly that caffeine is effective. Guaranine (which is nearly identical to caffeine) and the closely related alkaloids theobromine and theophylline make up the primary active agents in guarana. Caffeine's effects (and hence those of guaranine) are well known and include stimulating the central nervous system, increasing metabolic rate, and having a mild diuretic effect. Caffeine may have adverse effects on the blood vessels and other body systems, including dry mouth, headaches, and insomnia, and presumably guaranine would have similar effects.

Recommended dose: Since guarana is similar to caffeine, I don't recommend it for weight loss as there are other safer options. If you are going to use it for its stimulant effect, research shows 750 mg of guarana caps should be effective.

Yerba Maté

Yerba maté, also known as Paraguay tea, is a strong brain stimulant. Yerba maté contains more than 250 known natural compounds, most notably the alkaloids caffeine, theophylline, and theobromine. These agents promote central nervous stimulation, and act as diuretics, causing the body to shed water. Additionally, caffeine, theophylline, and theobromine appear to suppress appetite and boost metabolism. This makes yerba maté an ideal agent in the fight against unwanted fat.

Dried yerba maté naturally contains approximately one to two percent caffeine, yet some extracts may contain appreciably more natural caffeine. But most significant is the theobromine value of yerba maté's extracts. Like caffeine, theobromine is a central nervous system stimulant alkaloid, though it is appreciably weaker than caffeine. But theobromine is a stronger cardiac stimulant, smooth muscle relaxant, and diuretic. While dried yerba maté naturally contains approximately 0.45 to 0.9 percent theobromine, extracts may contain as much as 2 percent theobromine. This increase in theobromine gives yerba maté extracts unique diet properties.

Its weight loss effects are threefold, acting as an appetite suppressant, increasing your metabolism, and encouraging your body to burn more calories (a process called thermogenesis).

Recommended dose: 2 to 4 g cut leaves in 150 ml hot water (drink as a tea). In capsule form: 2 g once or twice per day.

Modulate Carbohydrate Metabolism

Many nutrients, including chromium and the B vitamins, are involved with the metabolism of carbohydrates. Nutrients that have this ability have been shown to increase insulin sensitivity and help lower high circulating insulin levels.

Chromium Picolinate

Chromium deficiency is associated with hyperglycemia, hyperinsulinemia, high triglycerides, and low levels of HDL. Chromium plays a role in carbohydrate and fat metabolism, potentially influencing weight and body composition.

Scientific research has not always been conclusively supportive of the appealing claims made about chromium's ability to aid weight loss. However, by helping to increase insulin sensitivity and to lower high insulin levels, chromium can aid in fat loss. Chromium has been shown to be an effective supplement to help reduce sugar cravings and suppress appetite—important elements in weight loss.

Recommended dosage: 400 to 600 mcg per day in the form of chromium picolinate.

Increase Fat Oxidation or Reduce Fat Synthesis

To lose weight in the form of fat, it is necessary to increase the rate of lipolysis (breakdown of fat) or increase the burning of fat. Losing weight in the form of fat is preferable because lean muscle mass will be maintained, and the fat loss will positively affect body composition, BMI, and body fat percentage.

L-carnitine

Fatty acids are the primary fuel source for adenosine triphosphate (ATP) production; however, they cannot cross the mitochondrial membrane without help. L-carnitine provides this help and acts as an energy transporter by shuttling fatty acids directly into the mitochondria to be burned as energy. According to a 2004 study in the *Journal Metabolism*, healthy adults can greatly enhance their fat-burning ability by supplementing with L-carnitine.

Recommended dosage: 500 mg to 2 grams per day.

Hydroxycitric Acid (HCA)

HCA is derived from the Malabar tamarind, a tropical fruit (*Garcinia cambogia*) native to India. HCA works by inhibiting the enzymes that convert carbohydrates into fat. If not utilized for energy, carbohydrates are converted into fat and stored in the body. HCA inhibits the conversion of carbohydrates into fat and promotes an increase in the formation of stored energy as glycogen. HCA also signals the brain to turn off hunger signals. New studies show that clinical strength doses of HCA increase fat oxidation ("burning"), as well as brain serotonin levels. Serotonin is a neurotransmitter involved in mood, sleep, and appetite control, and it may help address many of the emotional issues overweight people face, including binge eating and depression. No other HCA product has been shown to do this.

In a double-blind, placebo-controlled study, overweight subjects consuming hydroxycitric acid (HCA) demonstrated significantly greater weight loss than subjects consuming a placebo. The weight loss was primarily due to loss of fat. Appetite scores were reduced in the HCA group, but not in the placebo group. The group receiving HCA also had greater reductions in blood pressure, cholesterol levels, and hip and waist circumference than the group receiving the placebo. Test subjects received 1,320 mg HCA (in the form of CitriMax®) per day for 8 weeks.

Super CitriMax® is a highly bioavailable source of hydroxycitric acid (HCA) that is reported to decrease body weight. This study assessed the effects of Super CitriMax® on weight change and other variables in sixty moderately obese individuals. The subjects were randomly assigned to receive 4,667 mg Super CitriMax® (2,800 mg HCA) daily, or 4,667 mg Super CitriMax® combined with 400 mcg chromium (ChromeMate®) plus 400 mg *Gymnema sylvestre* extract, or a placebo. All three groups received a 2,000 Kcal diet and participated in supervised exercise. After eight weeks, both body weight and body mass index (BMI, an indicator of healthy body weight) decreased by 5 percent in the Super CitriMax® group. A 15.9 percent reduction in appetite (as measured by unconsumed food) was also observed, while urinary fat metabolites (a marker of fat breakdown) rose significantly. The Super CitriMax® group showed significant reductions in total cholesterol (7.2%), LDL cholesterol (13.2%), and triglycerides(5.9%). Additionally, levels of beneficial HDL increased by 3 percent. The combination group experienced even greater results in all areas tested. Only marginal or nonsignificant effects were observed in all test areas for the placebo group.

Recommended dose: 2.8 mg HCA per day.

Green Tea

Green tea has been used for thousands of years in Asia as both a beverage and a herbal medicine. Over the past few years, dozens of studies have been conducted on its antioxidative effect. Research has shown the beverage to be effective against a number of conditions, ranging from lowering cholesterol and capturing free radicals to reducing certain types of cancers.

A study published in the *American Journal of Clinical Nutrition* in 1999 showed that substances abundant in green tea extracts may promote weight loss. The study's participants were put on a typical Western diet of about 13 percent protein, 40 percent fat, and 47 percent carbohydrates. For six weeks, with each meal, the men took two capsules consisting of either green tea extract plus 50 mg caffeine, 50 mg of caffeine alone, or a placebo. Three times during the study, researchers measured the men's energy expenditure (EE, or the number of calories used in a 24-hour period) in a respiratory chamber. They also gauged the men's respiratory quotient or RQ (how well the body utilizes carbohydrates, protein, and fat). A lower RQ means that more fats are being metabolized by the body for energy.

The results showed that those men taking the green tea extract experienced a significant increase in 24-hour EE and a significant decrease in 24-hour RQ over those taking only caffeine or the placebo. Men taking the green tea extract also used more fat calories than those taking the placebo.

The scientists surmise that substances known as catechin polyphenols in the green tea extract may alter the body's use of norepinephrine, a chemical transmitter in the nervous system, to increase the rate of calorie burning. Green tea has thermogenic properties and promotes fat oxidation beyond that explained by its caffeine content. Green tea catechins can help prevent obesity by inhibiting the movement of glucose in fat cells. Epigallocatechin gallate (EGCG) has been found to be especially effective. There is now good evidence that green tea catechins are related to reductions in body fat.

Green tea is also an antioxidant and a useful blood sugar regulator, helping slow the rise of blood sugar after eating.

Recommended dose: Green tea can either be consumed as a tea beverage or taken in supplement form with standardized levels of EGCG. Consume 2 to 3 cups of tea per day. If you opt for the supplement, choose one that provides 90 mg ECCG; take three times per day before meals. The supplement forms are more effective for weight loss than the tea.

Conjugated Linoleic Acid (CLA)

CLA occurs naturally in dairy foods and grass-fed beef and lamb. It is produced by the intestinal bacteria of these animals when they convert omega-6 linoleic acid into CLA. Humans cannot convert linoleic acid into CLA, so we must rely on the foods we eat or supplementation to acquire the necessary amount of CLA. Unfortunately, the CLA content of dairy and meat products has declined over the last few decades because of increased antibiotic use in cattle and changes in the cattle's food supply from grass to grain.

Luckily, CLA is available today as a convenient dietary supplement, made by converting the high linoleic acid content of either sunflower or safflower oils into CLA. There are over 500 published studies supporting CLA's ability to exert positive effects on fat loss, prevent and control type 2 diabetes, protect against heart disease, reduce the risk of atherosclerosis, and modulate immune response.

The first human clinical trial using CLA was published in the *Journal of Nutrition* in 2000. The results showed that 3.5 g CLA per day showed a 20 percent reduction in body fat, with an average loss of seven pounds of fat.

Following that study, the effects of CLA on body composition of obese people were studied. Eighty overweight people took part in a six-month study in which they dieted and exercised. As expected, most initially lost weight, but once their diets ended, many regained some of their weight. The participants who were not given CLA put pounds back on in a fat-to-lean muscle mass ratio of 75 to 25, which is typical for most people. For those subjects taking CLA regularly, less fat was regained and more muscle mass retained, with an impressive, statistically significant ratio of 50 to 50.

Since CLA will help reduce body fat, and since reduced body fat improves insulin sensitivity, CLA has also demonstrated the ability to prevent and control type 2 diabetes by sensitizing insulin. Researchers from Purdue University in Indiana reported a dramatic improvement in serum insulin response in patients taking 6 g CLA daily. The eight-week clinical trial involved 22 subjects. More than 64 percent of the patients experienced an improvement in their leptin levels. (Leptin is the hormone that regulates both insulin and weight gain.) These results suggest that CLA can help prevent or delay the onset of diabetes.

Recommended dose: For weight loss, 3 g CLA isomers per day. Check the label as most CLA available is 60 to 70 concentration, meaning you would need to consume 4 to 5 g CLA to get 3 g CLA isomers. For improving insulin sensitivity, 6 CLA per day.

Coconut Oil (Medium-Chain Triglycerides)

All fats, whether they are saturated or unsaturated, contain the same number of calories. The medium-chain triglycerides (MCTs) in coconut oil, however, are different. They contain a little less because of the small size of the fatty acids, and they yield fewer calories than other fats. MCT, which is derived from coconut oil and consists of 75 percent caprylic acid and 25 percent capric acid, has an energy value of 6.8 calories per gram, unlike other fats, which yield 9 calories per gram.

The fat we eat is broken down into individual fats and repackaged into lipoproteins, which are sent into the bloodstream. The fatty acids are deposited directly into our fat cells. Other nutrients such as carbohydrates and protein are broken down and used immediately for energy or tissue building. Only when we eat too much is the excess carbohydrate converted into fat.

MCTs are digested and utilized differently. They are sent directly to the liver, where they are immediately converted into energy—just like a carbohydrate. So when you eat coconut oil, the body uses it immediately to make energy and does not store it as body fat.

MCTs also help increase your body's metabolic rate, which promotes weight loss. MCTs are easily absorbed and rapidly burned and used as energy for metabolism, thus increasing metabolic activity. MCTs can even help burn those other longer-chain fats you are consuming in your daily diet.

In one study, the fat-burning effect of a high-calorie diet containing 40 percent fat in the form of MCT was compared to a diet containing 40 percent fat in the form of long-chain fats (found in saturated fats). The thermogenic effect (metabolism) of the MCTs was almost twice as high as that of the long-chain fats; 120 calories versus 66 calories. The researchers concluded that the excess energy provided by fats in the form of MCTs would not be efficiently stored as fat, but rather would be burned.

Coconut oil contains the most concentrated source of MCTs available. Substituting coconut oil for other vegetable or cooking oils will help promote weight loss. Because of its fatty acid composition, coconut oil makes a great cooking oil—its fats are not destroyed by the high heat.

Not only is coconut oil great for cooking and weight loss, it is an incredible body moisturizer. I put coconut oil on my skin every day. It has been shown to prevent wrinkles, and it helps keep the skin hydrated and smelling delicious—good enough to eat!

Recommended dose: 2 to 4 tbsp coconut oil daily. Mix it in your protein smoothie, or add it into any recipe. For healthy, beautiful skin, smooth coconut oil over your entire body, and watch your skin radiate.

Pyruvate

Pyruvate is formed in the body during digestion of carbohydrates and protein from food. It may have a slight effect in helping you shed pounds, according to some studies. Pyruvate can be found in various foods, including red apples, cheese, and red wine.

Recommended dose: 1000 to 1500 mg per day and a calcium-rich diet.

Block Dietary Fat Absorption

Nutrients that can help to block the absorption of fat from your diet are similar to pharmaceutical drugs such as Xenical™ and Orlistat™. However, the nutrients do it in a natural way, with fewer side effects. The premise behind these nutrients is that because they cannot be digested, they pass through your gut where they bind with fat, thereby removing the fat from the body rather than allowing it to be absorbed.

Chitosan

Chitosan is made from chitin, a starch found in the skeletons of shrimp, crabs, and other shellfish. Chitosan cannot be digested, so it passes through your intestinal tract unabsorbed without adding any calories. The chemical nature of chitosan makes it bind with fatty foods, removing some of the fat from your body as it passes through rather than allowing the fat to be absorbed.

Five studies showed an average weight loss of 3.3 kg or 7 pounds over a placebo.

Recommended dose: 250 mg 2 to 3 times per day. For optimum results, take Chitosan with your two fattiest meals, which are usually lunch, dinner, or snacks for most people. It is important to drink at least 6 to 8 glasses of water a day, as the water assists the Chitosan in passing the fat through your digestive tract. The more water you drink, the better. You may also want to consider a vitamin C supplement to help stimulate the chitin in your bowel.

Increase Water Elimination

These herbs work as natural diuretics that increase the elimination of water from the body, which may result in significant weight loss. Many people retain a lot of fluid because they eat a high-salt diet, so this form of nutrient may be beneficial for water weight loss.

Dandelion

Dandelion is a natural diuretic, laxative, and digestive aid. It enhances fat metabolism; removes fatty acids and cholesterol from the bloodstream before they are stored in fat cells; and restores minerals lost when taking a diuretic. It may produce significant weight loss by decreasing body water.

Recommended dose: 3 to 4 cups tea (made from leaves, not roots) per day. Tincture: 15 to 30 drops per day. Or eat fresh dandelion greens in a soup or salad at meals.

Cascara

Cascara is a common ingredient used in weight-loss products. It is a strong stimulant, laxative and diuretic. Cascara is typically used in formulas with other digestive soothers such as marshmallow or chamomile.

Recommended dose: 500 to 1000 mg per day. In tea form, drink 1 to 2 cups per day. Tincture: 10 drops per day. Do not use cascara sagrada for more than a week at a time due to its strong laxative effect.

Enhance Mood

Certain hormones help us feel good. These are called serotonin-reuptake inhibitors. They work on the part of the brain that can control appetite, which leads to reduced calorie intake. This is especially beneficial for people who are emotional eaters.

St. John's Wort

A serotonin-reuptake inhibitor, it helps increase serotonin—our feel-good, happy hormone—levels, in the brain, and suppresses appetite, reduces depression-related overeating, and provides a feeling of fullness.

Recommended dose: 300 mg standardized extract with 0.3 percent hypericin 3 times per day. Tincture: 20 to 30 drops 3 times per day.

Miscellaneous

Guggul

Guggul is derived from the myrrh tree, a plant native to India. Guggul contains ketonic steroid compounds known as guggulsterones, which are believed to be responsible for guggul's cholesterol- and triglyceride-lowering actions. Studies show that guggul may also decrease platelet stickiness, thereby lowering the risk of coronary artery disease.

In some studies, guggul has been shown to increase the production of the thyroid hormone. Since this hormone is involved in the cell's breakdown of protein, fat, and carbohydrates, this herb will help promote weight loss.

Recommended dose: 25 mg guggulsterones three times per day.

Table 12.1: Summary of Supplements for Improved Insulin Response

Base supplements for everyone should include a whole-food multiple vitamin and 1 gram of omega-3 fatty acids from fish oil.(For specific brand recommendations please see the Product Resource Guide.)

Dosages based on current research recommendations. *Always check with your doctor before beginning any of these supplements.*

IR: Insulin Resistance
MS: Metabolic Syndrome
HD: Heart Disease Risk Factors (cholesterol, blood pressure, triglycerides)
Boldfacing indicates my recommendations based on the available research.

Continued

	Prevent IR	Treat IR	Treat MS	Treat Diabetes	Treat HD	Weight Loss	Increased Energy
Chromium	200 mcg	400–600 mcg	400–600 mcg	1000 mcg** Check with your physician if you are on oral hypoglycemic medications, as levels may need to be adjusted		400–600 mcg	
Biotin		9 mg		9 mg			
Zinc	30 mg	30 mg		30 mg		30–60 mg	
Magnesium	400 mg	400 mg		300–500 mg			
Vanadyl Sulfate				25–50 mg			
Fenugreek		5–15 g	5–15 g	5g x 3 per day	5g x 3 per day		
Vitamin B6				1.8 g	50 mg		
American Ginseng				3 g whole root			
Korean Ginseng				200 mg standardized extract or 0.5 to 2 g per day dry root			
Gymnema sylvestre		400 mg	400 mg	400 mg			
Cinnamon	1/2 tsp	1/2 tsp	1/2 tsp	1/2 tsp	1/2 tsp		1/2 tsp
Bitter melon				2 ounces of juice, 1500 mg capsules standardized to 2.5% bitters including charantins			

Table 12.2: Summary of Supplements for Improved Cholesterol/Lipid Levels

	Prevent IR	Treat IR	Treat MS	Treat Diabetes	Treat HD	Weight Loss	Energy
Omega-3*	1 g	1 g	1 g		2–3 g		
Vitamin B6					50mg		
Niacin					1.5–3 g		
Polymethoxylated Flavones*					300 mg		
Garlic (allicin)*					5000 mcg × 2 per day		
Beta Glucan*	1 g	2 g	2 g	2–3 g	3 g		
Fenugreek		5–15 g	5–15 g	5 g × 3 per day	5 g × 3 per day		

* Supplements I recommend before others.

Table 12.3: Summary of Antioxidants

	Prevent IR	Treat IR	Treat MS	Treat Diabetes	Treat HD	Weight Loss	Energy
Vitamin E	400 IU	800–1200 IU	800IU	800IU	2–3 g		
Vitamin C	500 mg	500 mg	500 mg	500–1000 mg	500–1000 mg		500 mg
CoQ 10*	60 mg	120 mg			120 mg		100 mg
Alpha Lipoic	50–300 mg	50–300 mg	50–300 mg	50–300 mg			

* Antioxidants I recommend before others.

Table 12.4: Summary of Supplements for Weight Loss

	Prevent IR	Treat IR	Treat MS	Treat Diabetes	Treat HD	Weight Loss	Energy
Glucomannan	Aim for 30 g of fiber per day	4 g	4 g		4 g	3 g x 3 times daily	
Hydroxy Citric Acid*			2.8 mg		2.8 mg	2.8 mg	
Yerba maté						2–4 g as a tea	
L-carnitine						500 mg–2 g	
Guarana						750 mg	
Calcium pyruvate	1000 mg	1500 mg				1500 mg	
Green tea				90 mg EGCG		90 mg EGCG	
Whey protein	25 g x 2 per day	25 g x 2 per day	25 g x 2 per day			25 g x 2 per day	
CLA*	6 g	6 g	3 g	6 g		3 g	
Coconut oil						2–4 tbsp	2 tbsp
Guggulsterones						25 mg x 3 per day	
Chitosan						250 mg 2–3 x daily	
Dandelion						3–4 cups tea 15–30 drops tincture	
Cascara						500–1000 mg	
St. John's wort*						300 mg standard-ized extract	
Chromium picolinate	200 mcg	400–600 mcg	400–800 mcg	1000 mcg		400–600 mcg	

* Supplements I recommend before others.

WHAT YOU HAVE LEARNED IN THIS CHAPTER

- There are many supplemental nutrients that can help prevent insulin resistance and metabolic syndrome by altering blood lipid levels, improving blood sugar levels, and/or helping you lose weight.
- A combination of a healthy diet, exercise, and supplements is your best approach. You cannot rely solely on supplements—it takes lifestyle changes to prevent and treat metabolic syndrome.
- Always consult with your health care provider before starting any supplement program.

Chapter 13

THE METABOLIC SYNDROME FOOD PROGRAM AND EATING TIPS

What you put in your mouth each day is the key to the prevention of insulin resistance, obesity, metabolic syndrome, diabetes, and heart disease, and in fact the list of conditions affected by your diet is far-reaching. You may need some help to get started on a lifetime of dietary changes. This chapter contains a five-day menu and plenty of recipes. You can choose the ones that fit your taste buds, desires, and lifestyle. Remember that your possibilities are endless, keeping in mind the principles you learned throughout the book. This chapter brings them all together in a range of options that incorporates low-GI carbohydrates, lean, nutritious sources of protein, and healthy fats, with plenty of vegetables.

DIETARY PRINCIPLES OF THE METABOLIC SYNDROME PROGRAM

1. Get in the habit of planning your meals in advance so you don't need to go to the grocery store every day.

2. Choose recipes that are easy and limit the use of expensive and difficult to find ingredients.

3. When buying raw vegetables, such as broccoli or cauliflower, cut them up and store them in plastic containers or large freezer bags, so they are ready and waiting for you to eat as a snack or to use in cooking.

4. Eat whole grains and low-GI carbohydrates.

5. Eat more wild fish and seafood rich in omega-3s.

6. Eat a protein with each meal and snack.

7. Incorporate whey protein powders twice per day, one mid-morning and one before dinner.

8. Eat five or six small meals per day.

9. Incorporate nutritional supplements into your day (see Chapter 12).

10. Make small changes to avoid overwhelming yourself. Small dietary changes will lead to a lifetime of healthy eating.

BREAKFAST MENUS AND RECIPES

Remember what your mother told you—she was right, breakfast is the most important meal of the day. Many people skip breakfast, or opt for the standard American breakfast of coffee and white toast. Although you think you may be doing your body a favor, or think that you are helping yourself lose weight, what you may be doing is promoting weight gain. When you don't eat for eight or nine hours (during the night when you are sleeping), your body goes into a fasting state in which you conserve and store more fat. If you eat first thing in the morning you will break this cycle, your metabolism will rev up again, and you will start burning calories more efficiently. This is the same concept as eating five or six small meals a day to keep your metabolism up and running so it does not go into starvation mode.

Here are some simple ideas for building a healthy and satisfying breakfast:

Protein Choices
- 2 eggs, poached, hard boiled, or scrambled
- 1 cup of plain yogurt
- 1 cup of nonfat, 1% or soy milk
- 2 tablespoons of peanut butter (use natural peanut butter or no trans fats options)
- 2 tablespoons of almond butter
- 2 ounces of cheese
- 1/2 cup of cottage cheese
- 1 small chicken breast
- 25 grams of whey protein powder
- Handful of nuts and seeds (try sunflower seeds, almonds, walnuts, hazelnuts)

Carbohydrate Choices
- 1 slice of whole wheat or rye toast
- 1/2 English muffin
- 1/2 cup of oatmeal
- 1/2 cup of multigrain cereal, for example Red River
- 1/2 cup of cold cereal rich in fiber and low in sugar
- 1 cup of berries
- 1 small whole wheat tortilla
- 1/2 banana (avoid bananas that are overripe)

Any of these protein and carbohydrate choices can be combined.

Day 1
Flax Berry Blast
1 scoop (25 g) low-carb whey protein
1 cup berries (fresh or frozen)
1/2 cup plain, low-fat, organic yogurt

1 tbsp ground flax seeds
1 tsp organic flax oil
1cup 1% milk or soy milk
Honey to taste

Place all ingredients in blender and blend until smooth.
You can modify recipe by changing type of fruit, milk beverage, or flavor of protein powder. I recommend a protein shake for breakfast at least 3 days a week.

1–2 servings

Per serving: 470 calories, 14 g fat, 44 g carbohydrates, 42 g protein

Day 2

Whole-grain cereal with nuts and yogurt

1 cup whole-grain cereal
1 tsp ground flax seeds
1 tsp chopped almonds and walnuts
1 cup plain nonfat yogurt
Honey to taste

1 serving

Per serving: 374 calories, 18 g fat, 33 g carbohydrates, 20 g protein

Day 3

1 cup oatmeal
1 tsp ground flax seeds
1/2 cup nonfat or 1% milk
Stevia or honey to taste
1/2 cup cottage cheese

1 serving

Per serving: 436 calories, 11 g fat, 71 g carbohydrates, 27 g protein

Day 4

2 poached eggs

1 slice whole-wheat toast

1 orange

> *1 serving*
>
> *Per serving: 219 calories, 11 g fat, 13 g carbohydrates, 17 g protein*

Day 5

Egg Frittata

1/2 cup chopped onions

1 clove garlic, minced

1 cup broccoli florets

1/2 cup chopped sweet red pepper

6 eggs

2 tbsp Parmesan cheese

1/4 cup shredded Cheddar cheese

3/4 tsp marjoram

1/4 tsp each salt and black pepper

Spray a pan with non-stick cooking spray. Add onions, garlic, broccoli, and red pepper. Cook over medium-high heat until tender-crisp, 4–5 minutes.

In a small bowl, combine eggs, Parmesan cheese, shredded cheese, marjoram, salt, and pepper. Mix well. Pour over vegetables. Tilt skillet to spread egg mixture evenly.

Reduce heat to medium-low. Cover and cook until set, about 10 minutes. Slide frittata onto a plate, then flip into skillet to brown opposite side (2–3 minutes).

> *2 servings*
>
> *Per serving: 220 calories, 5 g fat, 24 g carbohydrates, 21 g protein*

Day 6

1/2 cup cottage cheese

1 cup sliced fruit (strawberries)

1 slice whole-wheat toast

1 tbsp almond butter

> *1 serving*
>
> *Per serving: 372 calories, 12 g fat, 44 g carbohydrates, 22 g protein*

Day 7

Peanut Butter Banana Smoothie

25 g chocolate whey protein powder (reduced carbohydrate)

1 tbsp natural peanut butter

1/2 unripe banana

1 cup chocolate 1% milk

1 tbsp flax seeds

Ice cubes

Place all ingredients in blender and mix.

> *1–2 servings*
>
> *Per serving: 325 calories, 18 g fat, 35 g carbohydrates, 31 g protein*

LUNCH AND DINNER MENUS AND RECIPES

Keep in mind the dietary principles of the Metabolic Syndrome Program, and consume a whey protein shake mid-morning (before lunch) and one an hour before dinner. This will help keep your blood sugar levels balanced and prevent surges and spikes in insulin levels.

Also you need to remember that most vegetables are "free", meaning you can consume as many and as much of them as you want. Therefore, go ahead and eat cucumbers, tomatoes, or any other vegetable (with the exception of potatoes, carrots, and a few other choices—see the Appendix: Glycemic Index) as many times during the day as you like.

Day 1

Lunch

1 cup pasta salad (see recipe)

1/2 cup berries topped with 2 tbsp plain yogurt

Curried Salmon Pasta Salad

1 cup whole-wheat macaroni

8 oz canned salmon

1/2 cup minced red or yellow onion

1 cup diced celery

1 medium to large red apple, diced

1/2 cup chopped walnuts

Dressing

6 oz (3/4 cup) nonfat yogurt

2 tbsp olive oil

2 tsp fresh lemon juice

2 garlic cloves, crushed

1 tsp Dijon mustard

1/2 tsp salt, or to taste

Fresh ground black pepper to taste

Cook pasta per package directions; drain and rinse. In a large bowl, combine first six ingredients. In a small bowl, combine dressing ingredients. Pour dressing over salad; toss. Refrigerate, or serve at room temperature.

> *8 servings*
>
> *Per serving: 214 calories, 11 g fat, 18 g carbohydrate, 12 g protein*
>
> *Total menu: 334 calories, 13 g fat, 41 g carbohydrate, 18 g protein*

Dinner

Basil Chicken (see recipe)

1/2 cup cooked brown rice

Steamed broccoli
1 cup blueberries

Basil Chicken
4 skinless, boneless chicken breasts
1/2 small red onion
1/2 cup orange juice
1 tsp each dried basil, ground cumin
1/2 tsp salt
1/2 lime
1/4 cup coarsely chopped fresh basil

Lightly oil a large frying pan and set over medium heat. When hot, add chicken and cook until lightly golden. Meanwhile, thinly slice red onion. When chicken is golden, scatter onion around chicken. Pour in orange juice. Sprinkle with basil, cumin and salt.

Bring to a boil, then reduce heat to medium-low. Cover and simmer, turning chicken halfway through, 6–8 minutes. Squeeze lime juice over top. Remove chicken and place on dinner plates. Increase heat to high. Boil pan juices, stirring often, until slightly thickened, about 2 minutes. Stir in fresh basil. Drizzle over chicken. Serve with rice.

4 servings
Per serving: 187 calories, 7 g fat, 7 g carbohydrates, 22 g protein
Total menu: 429 calories, 9 g fat, 60 g carbohydrate, 27 g protein

Day 2
Lunch
Tuna Salad Wrap (see recipe)
Small mixed green salad
1/2 cup cottage cheese

Tuna Salad Wrap

1 can tuna packed in water
1 green onion, chopped
1/4 garlic clove, minced
1 celery stalk, chopped
1 tsp lemon juice
1 tbsp olive oil
Salt and pepper to taste
2 whole-wheat tortillas or pitas

Mix all ingredients except tortillas together and spread over tortillas or pitas.

2 servings

Per serving: 374 calories, 6 g fat, 45 g carbohydrates, 35 g protein

Mixed Green Salad

1 cup mixed field greens. Add 1/2 cup sliced cucumber, 1/2 cup tomato.

Healthy Dressing

1/2 cup olive oil
1/4 cup flaxseed oil
3 tbsp red wine vinegar
1 garlic clove, minced
1 tsp dry mustard
1 tsp Parmesan cheese
1 tbsp Italian herbs
Salt and pepper to taste

Place all ingredients in a shaker and shake. Pour over salad. If you refrigerate the dressing, take it out of the fridge at least one hour before using, so the olive oil has a chance to settle.

Total menu: 635 calories, 15 g fat, 74 g carbohydrates, 51 g protein

Dinner

Vegetarian Chili (see recipe)

1 whole-wheat dinner roll

1 cup berries (top with 1/2 cup lemon yogurt)

Chili Chili Bang Bang

Recipe courtesy of *LooneySpoons*

Non-stick cooking spray

1 1/4 cup coarsely chopped onions

1 cup each chopped sweet green and red pepper

3/4 cup each chopped celery and carrot

3 cloves garlic, minced

1 tbsp chili powder

1 1/2 cups quartered mushrooms

1 cup cubed zucchini

1 can (28 oz) tomatoes, undrained, cut up

1 can (19 oz) black beans, drained and rinsed

1 can (19 oz) chickpeas, drained and rinsed

1 can (12 oz) kernel corn, undrained

1 tbsp ground cumin

1 1/2 tsp each dried oregano, basil

1/2 tsp cayenne pepper, ort to taste

Spray a large frying pan with non-stick cooking spray. Add onions, green and red peppers, celery, carrots, garlic, and chili powder. Cook over medium heat, stirring often, until vegetables are softened.

Add mushrooms and zucchini. Cook, stirring, for 4 more minutes. Add tomatoes, beans, chickpeas, corn (with liquid), cumin, oregano, basil, and cayenne pepper. Stir well. Bring to a boil. Reduce heat to medium-low. Cover and simmer for 20 minutes, stirring occasionally.

8 servings

Per serving: 190 calories, 2 g fat, 38 g carbohydrate, 9 g protein

Total menu: 544 calories, 8g fat, 77 g carbohydrate, 26 g protein

Day 3

Lunch

Turkey Barley Soup

1/2 cup mixed green salad

Turkey Barley Soup

Recipe courtesy of *LooneySpoons*

2 tsp oil

1 lb skinless turkey breasts, cut into cubes

1 1/2 cups each chopped celery and carrot

1 cup chopped onions

4 cups low-sodium, reduced-fat chicken broth

1 can (28 oz) tomatoes, undrained, cut up

1/3 cup pearl barley

3/4 tsp dried marjoram

1/2 tsp each ground thyme, sage, salt, and black pepper

1/4 cup chopped fresh parsley

Heat oil in a large saucepan over medium-high heat. Add turkey cubes and cook until no longer pink.

Add all remaining ingredients. Mix well. Bring soup to a boil over high heat. Reduce heat to low. Cover and simmer for 30–35 minutes, until turkey and barley are tender.

6 servings

Per serving: 257 calories, 5 g fat, 25 g carbohydrate, 27 g protein

Total menu: 390 calories, 10 g fat, 45 g carbohydrate, 30 g protein

Dinner

Dill Salmon

1/2 cup cooked wild rice

Grilled asparagus

1 cup berries

Dill Salmon

1/2 cup low-fat sour cream

2 tsp horseradish

Juice of 1/2 lemon

1/2 tsp dried dill weed

1/4 tsp black pepper

1/2 cup unseasoned whole-wheat dry bread crumbs

2 tbsp Parmesan cheese

3/4 tsp dried oregano

1/4 tsp paprika

4 salmon fillets

1 egg, well beaten

Preheat oven to 425°

To prepare dill sauce, combine sour cream, horseradish, lemon juice, dill weed, and pepper in a small bowl. Cover and refrigerate until ready to serve.

To prepare bread crumb coating, mix bread crumbs, cheese, oregano, and paprika in a small bowl. Spread mixture evenly on a dinner-size plate.

Rinse fish and pat dry. Dip fish in egg, then crumb coating. Coat both sides.

Place fish in a shallow baking pan sprayed with non-stick cooking oil. Cook, 10 minutes per 1 inch of thickness. Remove from pan and spoon dill sauce over top. Serve with rice.

4 servings

Per serving: 243 calories, 5 g fat, 15 g carbohydrates, 34 g protein

Total menu: 413 calories, 5 g fat, 49 g carbohydrates, 43 g protein

Day 4

Lunch

Sesame Chicken Salad

2 cups cooked whole-wheat pasta (try rotini)

2 cups chopped cooked chicken breast

1 cup each thinly sliced sweet red pepper and broccoli florets

1 cup snow peas, trimmed and halved

1/4 cup chopped green onions

3 tbsp red wine vinegar

1 tbsp reduced-sodium soy sauce

2 tbsp tomato-based chili sauce

2 tsp sesame oil

1 tsp grated gingerroot

1 tsp honey

1 clove garlic, minced

1/4 tsp black pepper

In a large bowl, toss cooked pasta with chicken, red pepper, broccoli, snow peas, and green onions. Set aside.

In a small bowl, whisk together vinegar, soy sauce, chili sauce, sesame oil, gingerroot, honey, garlic, and pepper.

Pour dressing over pasta mixture and stir to coat evenly. Refrigerate until ready to serve.

2–3 servings

Per serving: 120 calories, 4 g fat, 12 g carbohydrate, 11 g protein

Dinner

Stir-Fry Vegetables and Tofu in Peanut Sauce (recipe below)

1 cup cooked brown rice

1 cup berries

Stir-Fry Vegetables and Tofu in Peanut Sauce

1 (10 1/2) oz package firm tofu

1/4 cup soy sauce

Non-stick spray oil

1 large onion, cut into wedges

1 lb fresh or frozen stir-fry vegetables

1/2 cup chicken broth

1 tbsp peanut butter

1/4 cup vinegar

3 tbsp soy sauce

1/4 tsp cayenne pepper

1/4 tsp ground ginger

4 cloves garlic, minced

2 tsp cornstarch

Drain and rinse tofu. Slice into 1/2 inch cubes. Marinate in soy sauce. Meanwhile, coat a non-stick pan or wok with spray oil. Brown onion in pan. Add stir-fry vegetables. Cover and steam until almost tender. Pour into serving bowl and set aside.

Wipe pan. Spray again with oil. Drain tofu. Heat pan, add tofu, and cook, turning pieces gently, until browned. Add vegetables. In a separate bowl, combine chicken broth, peanut butter, vinegar, soy sauce, cayenne, ginger, garlic, and cornstarch. Add to tofu and vegetables. Cook, stirring often, until sauce is clear and bubbly.

6 servings

Per serving: 173 calories, 8 g fat, 11 g carbohydrates, 14 g protein

Total menu: 440 calories, 10 g fat, 67 g carbohydrates, 20 g protein

Day 5

Lunch

Strawberry Spinach Salad

12 oz raw spinach, torn into bite-sized pieces

1 cup fresh sliced strawberries

1/4 cup slivered almonds

Dressing

1/2 cup olive oil

1 tsp stevia

2 tsp salt

2 tbsp poppy seeds

1/2 cup white wine vinegar

>*4 servings*
>
>*Per serving: 487 calories, 35 g fat, 42 g carbohydrates, 6 g protein*

Dinner

1/2 rotisserie-chicken or roasted chicken (skin removed)

Steamed broccoli and cauliflower

1/2 cup brown rice

>*Per serving: 501 calories, 36 g fat, 3 g carbohydrate, 40 g protein*
>
>*Total menu: 640 calories, 37 g fat, 29 g carbohydrate, 45 g protein*

Day 6

Lunch

Chicken Salad with Thai-Flavored Dressing

3 cups shredded rotisserie chicken (use last night's leftovers)

2 medium celery stalks, diced

2 medium green onions, sliced thin

1/4 cup chopped honey-roasted peanuts

2 tbsp lime juice

2 tbsp Asian fish sauce

1 tsp ground ginger

2 tsp sugar

1/2 tsp hot red pepper flakes

2 tbsp each minced fresh cilantro, mint

Green leaf lettuce

Sliced cucumbers

Grated carrot

Extra chopped peanuts

In a medium bowl, mix chicken, celery, green onions, and peanuts. In a small bowl, whisk lime juice, fish sauce, ginger, sugar, red pepper, cilantro, and mint with 2 tbsp water. Toss dressing with chicken mixture and serve on a bed of green leaf lettuce, with sliced cucumbers, grated carrots, and extra chopped peanuts.

4 servings

Per serving: 326 calories, 17 g fat, 10 g carbohydrates, 38 g protein

Dinner

Beef and Red Bean Enchiladas (recipe below)

1/2 cup mixed greens (add cucumbers, tomatoes)

1 tbsp Healthy Dressing (Day 2)

Beef and Red Bean Enchiladas

1 pound extra lean ground beef

1 can (15 1/2 oz) of small red or pinto beans, drained

2 cups grated pepper Jack cheese

1 medium onion

2 tbsp olive oil

1 can (15 oz) tomato sauce

1 can (14 1/4 oz) chicken broth

3 tbsp sour cream

12 corn tortillas

Optional garnish: chopped fresh cilantro, hot red pepper sauce

Heat oven to 375°. In a pan, brown the ground beef. In a medium bowl, mix together browned beef, beans, and 1 cup cheese; set aside. Thinly slice 1/2 cup onion; set aside. Finely chop remaining onion. Heat oil in a 12-inch skillet over medium-high heat. Add chopped onions and sauté until golden, about 5 minutes, stirring frequently; reduce heat if sputtering. Add broth; bring to simmer. Remove from heat; whisk in sour cream. Stir 1/2 cup sauce into beef mixture. Spread 1/2 cup sauce in a 13-by-9 inch ovenproof glass dish. Microwave tortillas on high power in a microwave-safe plastic bag until warm, about 1 minute. Fill each tortilla with a heaping 1/4 cup beef mixture; roll and place in baking dish. Top with remaining sauce and cheese. Bake until bubbly, about 20 minutes. Top with sliced onions and cilantro and pepper sauce, if desired. Serve hot.

   6 servings

   Per serving: 550 calories, 30 g fat, 45 g carbohydrates, 25 g protein

   Total menu: 623 calories, 35 g fat, 52 g carbohydrates, 25 g protein

Day 7

Lunch

Low Fat Broccoli Soup (recipe below)

1/2 cup mixed green salad with cucumber, tomato, shredded carrots, and 1 tbsp Healthy Dressing (Day 2)

1/2 cup mixed berries with a dollop of vanilla yogurt

Low Fat Broccoli Soup

Recipe courtesy of *LooneySpoons*

1 cup chopped onions

1 clove garlic, minced

1/2 cup chopped celery

2 1/2 cups low-sodium, reduced-fat chicken broth

3 cups broccoli florets

1 cup peeled, cubed potato

1/2 cup low-fat sour cream

3/4 cup shredded reduced-fat sharp Cheddar cheese

1/2 tsp each ground thyme, black pepper, and lite Worcestershire sauce

1/4 tsp salt

4–5 dashes hot pepper sauce

Spray a large saucepan with non-stick spray. Add onions, garlic, and celery. Cook, stirring, over medium heat until celery begins to soften, about 5 minutes. Add broth, 2 cups broccoli, and potato. Bring to a boil. Reduce heat to medium-low. Cover and simmer for 10–12 minutes until broccoli and potatoes are tender.

While soup is simmering, steam reserved 1 cup broccoli until tender, about 5 minutes. Set aside.

Transfer soup to a blender or food processor, working in batches if necessary. Pulse on and off until soup is coarsely pureed. Return pureed soup to pot and place over low heat. Add reserved steamed broccoli, sour cream, cheese, thyme, pepper, Worcestershire sauce, salt, and hot pepper sauce. Stir until smooth.

4–6 servings

Per serving: 109 calories, 3g fat, 13 g carbohydrates, 9 g protein

Total menu: 259 calories, 7 g fat, 39 g carbohydrate, 10 g protein

Dinner

Lemon Broiled Sole (recipe below)

3/4 cup baked sweet potato

1 cup grilled zucchini

Lemon Broiled Sole

1 1/4 lb sole fillet

2 tbsp fresh lemon juice

1 tbsp brown sugar

1 tbsp olive oil

Rinse fish with cold water and pat dry with a paper towel. Cut fish into four pieces and place in a shallow baking dish.

Combine lemon juice, brown sugar, and oil in a small bowl. Drizzle lemon mixture over fish, turning so both sides are coated with marinade. Cover and marinate in the refrigerator for 15 minutes.

Preheat oven broiler. Transfer fish to broiler pan coated with vegetable oil spray. Broil 3–6 minutes (depending on thickness), then turn, baste with remaining marinade, and broil until fish flakes easily with a fork.

Guideline: cook fish for a total of 10 minutes per inch of thickness.
4 servings
Per serving: 169 calories, 5 g fat, 3 g carbohydrate, 27 g protein
Total menu: 349 calories, 5 g fat, 44 g carbohydrate, 32 g protein

These sample menus and recipes will help get you started on the road to long-term dietary changes. The recipes are easy to make and utilize everyday ingredients. You can make some of the recipes on the weekend and freeze them—chilies and soups freeze well and can be thawed the night before serving. Many of the recipes make more than one serving, and are great the next day as leftovers. Keep in mind the ten dietary principles of the Metabolic Syndrome Program, and you will be on your way to healthy eating, weight loss, and prevention and treatment of metabolic syndrome. Also, a positive attitude goes a long way in achieving your goals.

A respected doctor, colleague, and friend once told me, "Give yourself the proper nutrients, and you are on your way to health."

WHAT YOU HAVE LEARNED IN THIS CHAPTER

- Healthy food choices are the key to disease prevention.
- Eat five or six small meals a day. Consume a protein shake two times daily, one mid-morning and one before dinner.
- Variety is the spice of life. Give new recipes a try.

Appendix

GLYCEMIC INDEX

For further information on the glycemic index, visit www.mendosa.com

LOW-GLYCEMIC FOODS: RATED 55 OR LESS (YOUR BEST OPTIONS)

Fruits

All berries, 1 cup	Kiwifruit, 1 medium	Grapes, 1 cup
Cherries, 10 large	Pear, 1 medium	Mango, 1 small
Apple, 1 medium	Plums, 1 medium	Unripe banana, 1 medium
Orange, 1 medium	Grapefruit, 1/2 medium	
Peach, 1 medium	Prunes, pitted, 6	

Vegetables

Artichokes, 1 cup	Yam, boiled, 3 oz
Asparagus, 1 cup	Kale, cooked, 1 cup; raw, 2 cups
Bell peppers, 1 cup, cooked or raw	Spinach, cooked, 1 cup; raw, 2 cups
Broccoli, 1 cup	Tomato, 1 medium
Cabbage, cooked or raw, 1 cup	Zucchini, cooked or raw, 1 cup
Tomato soup, canned, 1 cup	Cauliflower, 1 cup
Sweet potatoes, mashed 1/2 cup	Carrots, boiled, raw, 1/2 cup
Eggplant, 1 cup	Corn on the cob, boiled, 80 g
Brussels sprouts, 1 cup	or medium sized
Carrots, raw, boiled, canned, 1/2 cup	

Cereals/Grains

All Bran, 1 tbsp	Cappelini pasta, cooked, 1 cup
Oatmeal, 1 cup	Brown rice, cooked, 1 cup
Whole-grain pastas, cooked, 1 cup	Buckwheat, cooked, 1/2 cup, 80 g
Pearl barley, 1/2 cup	Tortellini, with cheese, cooked, 180 g
Bran Buds, 1 tbsp	Ravioli, meat-filled, cooked, 1 cup, 30 g
Rice bran, 1 tbsp	Vermicelli, cooked, 1 cup, 180 g
Muesli, natural	Spaghetti, 1 cup, 180 g
Bulgur, cooked, 1/2 cup	Fettuccini, cooked, 1 cup, 180 g
Sourdough bread, 1 slice	Star pastina, cooked, 1 cup, 180 g

Beans/Legumes

Adzuki beans, 1/2 cup	Navy beans, boiled, 1/2 cup
Butter beans, 1/2 cup	Pinto beans, soaked, boiled, 1/2 cup
Black beans, 1/2 cup	Soy, boiled, 1/2 cup
Garbanzo beans, 1/2 cup	Chickpeas, 1/2 cup
Kidney beans, 1/2 cup	Lima beans, cooked, 1/2 cup
Split peas, boiled, 1/2 cup	Baked beans, canned in tomato sauce, 1/2 cup
Lentils, 1/4 cup	Unsalted peanuts, 1/2 cup
Lima beans, 1/2 cup	

Sweeteners/Miscellaneous

Stevia	Strawberry jam, 1 tbsp
FOS (Fructo-oligosaccharides)	Fructose, 2 tsp
Dark Chocolate (more than 60% cocoa)	Corn chips, Doritos, Original, 50 g

Dairy

Plain yogurt, 1 cup	Custard, 1/2 cup
Soy beverages, 1 cup	Organic milk, skim, 1%, 2%, or whole), 1 cup
Chocolate milk, 1 cup	

Beverages

Apple juice, unsweetened, 1 cup	Orange juice, unsweetened, 1 cup
Grapefruit juice, unsweetened, 1 cup	Pineapple juice, unsweetened, 1 cup

MODERATE-GLYCEMIC FOODS: RATED 56 TO 69 (LIMITED CONSUMPTION)

Fruits

Raisins, 1/4 cup	Apricots, 3 medium
Pineapple, fresh, 2 slices, 125 g	Cantaloupe, 1/4 small
Figs, dried, 50 g	Papaya, 1/2 medium
Bananas (semi-hard), 1 medium	

Vegetables/Legumes

Beets, 1/4 cup	Gnocchi, cooked, 1 cup
Cornmeal, 1/3 cup	

Grains

Basmati rice, cooked, 1 cup	Pita, 1 piece, 65 g
Long grain white rice, cooked, 1 cup	Popcorn, popped, 2 cups
Wild rice, 1 cup	Whole-grain bread, 1 slice
Millet, cooked, 1/2 cup	Pumpernickel bread, 1 slice
Couscous, 2/3 cup	Rye bread, 1 slice
Cornmeal, 1/3 cup	Hamburger or hot dog bun, prepackaged, 1
Macaroni and cheese, packaged, cooked, 220 g	Croissant, 1, 50 g

Breakfast Cereals

Bran, 1/2 cup	Weet-Bix, 2 biscuits, 30 g
Shredded Wheat, 1/3 cup, 25 g	Just Right, 3/4 cup, 30 g
Mini-Wheats (whole wheat), 1 cup, 30 g	Just Right Just Grains, 1 cup, 45 g

Crackers

Breton Wheat Crackers, 6, 25 g	Stoned Wheat Thins, 5, 25 g
Ryvita, 2, 20 g	

Beverages

Soft drink, 1 can	Cranberry juice, cocktail, 1 cup
Strawberry Nestle Quick, 3 tsp	

Sweeteners/Misc

Unrefined raw honey, 1 tbsp

Organic unrefined brown sugar, 2 tsp

Vanilla ice cream, 1/2 cup

White sugar, 2 tsp

Muffins, apricot, coconut,
    and honey, from mix, 50 g

Muffins, banana, oat, and honey,
    from mix, 50 g

Muffin, bran, 1, 80 g

Muffin, blueberry, 1, 80 g

HIGH-GLYCEMIC FOODS: RATED 70-100 (EAT AS A TREAT ON OCCASION)

Fruits

Most dried fruits

Ripe bananas

Dates, dried, 5

Watermelon, 1 cup

Vegetables/Legumes

Parsnips, boiled, 1/2 cup

Red potato, baked, 4 oz, 1 medium

Red potato, skinned, boiled, 4 oz, 1 medium

Potatoes, mashed, 1/2 cup

Pumpkin, peeled, boiled, 1/2 cup

French Fries, fine cut, 120 g

Grains

White bread, 1 slice

French bread, 1 slice

Whole wheat bread, 1 slice

Bagel, 1/2

French baguette, 1 oz, 30 g

Rice pasta, brown, cooked, 1 cup, 180 g

Breakfast Cereals

Cheerios, 1/2 cup, 30 g

Corn bran, 1/2 cup, 30 g

Wheatbites, 30 g

Total, 30 g

Puffed Wheat, 1 cup, 30g

Bran flakes, 3/4 cup, 30 g

Froot Loops, 1 cup

Cocoa Puffs, 3/4 cup, 30 g

Corn Chex, 30 g

Corn Flakes, 1 cup, 30 g

Rice Krispies, 1 cup, 30 g

Grape-Nuts, 1/2 cup, 58 g

Raisin Bran, 1 cup, 45 g

Beverages

Soft drink, 1 cup	Gatorade, 1 cup

Crackers

Premium soda crackers, 3, 25 g	Crackers, graham, 1, 30 g
Rice cakes, 2, 25 g	Water crackers, 5, 25 g

Sweeteners

Corn syrup solids, 2 tsp	High fructose corn syrup, 2 tsp
Maltose, 2 tsp	Glucose, 2 tsp

Snack Foods

Pretzels, 50 g	Scones, made from packet mix, 1 scone, 40 g
Skittles, 62 g	Tofu Frozen Dessert (nondairy), 100 g
Corn chips, 1 oz	

RESOURCE GUIDE

Nature's Way
10 Mountain Springs Parkway
Springville, UT   84663
1-800-926-8883
www.naturesway.com

Sweet Leaf Stevia
2546 W Birchwood Avenue
Suite 104
Mesa, AZ   85202
1-800-899-9908
www.sweetleaf.com

Cevena BioProducts Inc.
Research Transition Facility
8308-114 Street
Edmonton, AB   T6G 2E1
www.cevena.com

Nutrition 21
4 Manhattanville Road
Suite 202
Purchase, NY   10577
www.diachrome.com

INFORMATIONAL WEBSITES

www.karlenekarst.com

www.doctormurray.com

www.fatsforhealth.com

www.supplementinfo.org

www.medicinenet.com

www.diabetes.ca

www.dietitians.ca

www.heartandstroke.com

www.mercola.com

RECOMMENDED READING

Healthy Fats for Life
By Lorna Vanderhaeghe and Karlene Karst
(Toronto: John Wiley & Sons, 2004)

How to Prevent and Treat Diabetes with Natural Medicine
By Dr. Michael Murray and Michael Lyon
(New York: Riverhead Books, 2003)

The Encyclopedia of Healing Foods
By Dr. Michael Murray
(New York: Atria Books, 2005)

The Food Connection
By Sam Graci
(Toronto: Macmillan Canada, 2001)

The Omega-3 Connection
By Dr. Andrew Stoll
(New York: Simon & Schuster, 2001)

The Inflammation Nation
By Dr. Floyd Chilton
(New York: Simon & Schuster, 2005)

The Coconut Oil Miracle
By Dr. Bruce Fife
(New York: Avery Books, 2004)

Syndrome X
By Jack Challem, Burton Berkson, and Melissa Smith
(Toronto: John Wiley & Sons, 2000)

Diabesity
By Dr. Francine Kaufman
(New York: Bantam Books, 2005)

RECOMMENDED COOKBOOKS

Cook Great Food
By Dietitians of Canada
(Toronto: Robert Rose Inc., 2001)

Rebar
Modernfoodcookbook
By Audrey Alsterberg and Wanda Urbanowicz
(Victoria: Bigideaspublishinginc, 2001)

LooneySpoons
By Janet and Greta Podleski
(Ottawa: Granet Publishing Inc., 1996)

Eat, Shrink & Be Merry
By Janet and Greta Podleski
(Ottawa: Granet Publishing Inc, 2005)

GLOSSARY OF TERMS

Alpha Linolenic Acid (ALA): Is the parent omega-3 polyunsaturated fatty acid. ALA is the precursor to eicosapentaenoic acid (EPA) and docosahexaenoic acid (DHA).

Amino Acids: The building blocks of protein. There are twenty amino acids in total. Twelve are nonessential, meaning our body can make them; eight are essential, meaning they must be supplied by our diet.

Arachidonic Acid (AA): Is an omega-6 polyunsaturated fatty acid. Arachidonic acid is abundant in the diet, and is found in eggs as well as animal and fish fats. AA is the precursor to hormones, including prostaglandins series 2 and leukotrienes series 4. It has varied effects, including blood vessel constriction and pro-inflammatory effects.

Body Mass Index (BMI): According to the World Health Organization, this is the best way to determine if you are overweight or obese. It is defined as weight in kilograms divided by the square of your height in meters.

Branched-chain amino acids (BCAAs): Include leucine, isoleucine, and valine, and are important for athletes since unlike the other essential amino acids, they are metabolized directly into muscle tissue and are the first ones used during exercise and resistance training. Whey protein is an excellent source of the BCAA leucine.

Carbohydrates: Are chemical compounds that contain oxygen, hydrogen, and carbon atoms. They consist of monosaccharide sugars of varying chain lengths. They are classified by the number of sugar units into monosaccharides (such as glucose), disaccharides (such as saccarose), oligosaccharides (such as fructooligosaccharide), and polysaccharides (such as starch, glycogen, and cellulose).

Conjugated Linoleic Acid (CLA): Is a polyunsaturated fatty acid with one of the double bonds in the cis position and the other in the trans configuration. The most common natural CLA is the cis-9 and trans-11. CLA is converted through a patented process from linoleic acid, which is found in high concentrations in sunflower and safflower oils.

C-Reactive Protein (CRP): Is a blood protein produced by the liver. CRP levels rise dramatically during the inflammatory phase, and it is used mainly as a marker of inflammation.

Cytokines: Proteins that are released by the immune system and promote inflammation.

Docosahexaenoic Acid (DHA): Is an omega-3 polyunsaturated fatty acid. DHA is a very long-chain fatty acid formed in the body through a series of steps, starting with ALA. DHA is used in membranes, especially in the brain and eye.

Eicosanoids: Are a family of powerful, hormone-like compounds produced from EFAs. Eicosanoids include prostaglandins, leukotrtienes, and thromboxanes, which are responsible for many of the beneficial effects of EFAs. Eicosanoids control numerous body processes (for example, inflammation, blood clotting, blood pressure, and immune response) and are formed in the body from essential fatty acids.

Eicosapentaenoic Acid (EPA): An omega-3 polyunsaturated fatty acid. EPA is a very long-chain fatty acid formed from ALA through a series of steps. EPA is the immediate precursor to beneficial hormones that have anti-inflammatory and blood-thinning effects.

Fiber: The portion of the plant that cannot be digested by the human digestive tract. It is classified as soluble and insoluble.

Free radicals: Are molecules with unpaired electrons, which are highly reactive. Free radicals are a leading cause of chronic disease.

Gamma Linolenic Acid (GLA): Is an omega-6 polyunsaturated fatty acid that can be formed by linoleic acid. It has very potent anti-inflammatory effects. It is not common in the diet, but can be found in highest concentrations in borage and evening primrose oil.

Ghrelin: A powerful appetite-stimulating hormone.

Glucagon: A hormone secreted by the pancreas. Glucagon's job is to release stored glucose from the liver into the bloodstream.

Glucose: The simple sugar that is the main source of fuel for the body.

Glycemic Index: A numerical index given to a carbohydrate-rich food that is based on the average increase in blood glucose levels after the food is eaten.

Glycemic Load: Is a ranking system for carbohydrate content in foods based on their glycemic index. It is calculated as the quantity of carbohydrate (content in grams) multiplied by its GI and divided by 100. For example, a 100 g slice of watermelon with a GI of 72 and a carbohydrate content of 5 g (it contains a lot of water) makes the calculation $5 \times 0.72 = 3.6$, the GL is 3.6. So a food with a GI of 100 and a carbohydrate content of 10 g has a GL of 10 ($10 \times 1 = 10$), while a food with 100 g carbohydrate and a GI of just 10 also has a GL of 10 ($100 \times 0.1 = 10$).

Hemoglobin A1c (HbA1c): A measure of long-term blood glucose levels. Diabetics need to aim for an HbA1c level of less than 7%, which indicates good blood sugar control.

High-Density Lipoprotein (HDL): Is the blood lipoprotein that contains high levels of protein and low levels of cholesterol, and is the most dense of the lipoproteins. Synthesized primarily in the liver and small intestine, HDL picks up cholesterol and transfers it to other lipoproteins. HDL cholesterol is known as "good cholesterol" as it helps carry cholesterol away from the heart to the liver to be excreted, and therefore lowers the risk of coronary heart disease. Low levels of HDL are a component of metabolic syndrome.

Hyperglycemia: Is too high a level of glucose (sugar) in the blood; this can be a sign that diabetes is out of control. Many things can cause hyperglycemia. It occurs when the body does not have enough insulin or cannot use the insulin it does have to turn glucose into energy. Some signs of hyperglycemia can be a dry mouth, being very thirsty, and a need to urinate often.

Hypertension: Also known as high blood pressure (blood pressure that is consistently—for more than 6 months—above 140/90). Systolic blood pressure is the top number. Diastolic blood pressure is the bottom number. Hypertension may have no known cause (essential or idiopathic hypertension) or be associated with other primary diseases (secondary hypertension). Hypertension is a component of metabolic syndrome and increases your risk of developing cardiovascular disease.

Hypoglycemia: Abnormally low blood sugar levels. Hypoglycemia usually occurs when the pancreas oversecretes insulin; symptoms may indicate diabetes and include jitteriness, rapid breathing, and lethargy.

Impaired Fasting Glucose: Blood sugar levels that are higher than normal during fasting, but not high enough to be diabetes. This is known as prediabetes and is a component of metabolic syndrome.

Impaired Glucose Tolerance: A condition associated with excessive elevation in blood sugar after a meal, but not meeting the criteria for a diagnosis of diabetes.

Inflammation: Is the first response of the immune system to infection or irritation. It is characterized by redness, heat, swelling, pain, and dysfunction of organs involved.

Insoluble Fiber: Speeds up intestinal transit time, helping sweep the colon and improving regularity. Insoluble fiber is found in wheat bran, whole-grain products, and vegetables, as well as flax seeds.

Insulin Resistance: A condition in which the cells no longer respond well to insulin. As a result, the body secretes more insulin into the bloodstream in an effort to reduce blood glucose levels.

Leptin: A hormone that suppresses appetite.

Linoleic Acid (LA): Is an omega-6 polyunsaturated fatty acid found in abundance in the average diet (in vegetable oils, margarine, and processed foods). We get too much LA in our diet, which has created numerous health problems, especially those related to inflammation.

Low-Density Lipoprotein (LDL): Is the blood lipoprotein that contains low levels of protein and high levels of cholesterol. As LDL circulates in the blood, it can slowly build up in the walls of the arteries that feed the heart and brain, and may result in hardening of the arteries. LDL is often referred to as "bad cholesterol" because it carries cholesterol to the heart, and therefore increases the risk of heart disease.

Metabolic Syndrome: A constellation of multiple metabolic risk factors caused by or related to insulin resistance. These include high triglyceridesTG levels, a low HDL-C level, high blood pressure, glucose intolerance, obesity, and increased inflammatory markers.

Omega-3: Is the term for the polyunsaturated fatty acids, including ALA, EPA, and DHA.

Omega-6: Is the term for the polyunsaturated fatty acids, including LA, GLA, and AA.

Pedometer: Senses your body's motion and counts your footsteps. This count is converted into distance by knowing the length of your usual stride. Wear a pedometer every day to record the total number of steps you take. Aim for 10,000 steps per day.

Prediabetes: Elevated blood glucose levels below the threshold for diabetes that have clinical consequences. The term "prediabetes" is a practical and convenient term for impaired fasting glucose and impaired glucose tolerance, which places individuals at risk of developing diabetes and its complications.

Proteins: Are essential components of the body that are required for its structure and proper function. Proteins function as enzymes, hormones, and antibodies, as well as transport and structural components. They are made of building blocks called amino acids.

Soluble Fiber: Delays the time of transit through the intestine to provide a sponge-like action. Soluble fiber is useful in removing toxins and in lowering cholesterol and blood sugar. It can be found in oats, beans, dried peas, and legumes, as well as flax seeds.

Triglycerides: Are composed of three fatty acids attached to a glycerol backbone. Most dietary fats are consumed in the form of triglycerides. Triglycerides are the predominant storage form of fat in the body. High triglycerides are a component of metabolic syndrome.

Type 1 Diabetes: Diabetes that is primarily a result of pancreatic beta cell destruction and that is prone to ketoacidosis. This form includes diabetes caused by an autoimmune process and diabetes for which the cause of the beta cell destruction is unknown. It is diagnosed with a fasting blood glucose level of >/- 7.0 mmol/L.

Type 2 Diabetes: May range from predominant insulin resistance with relative insulin deficiency to a predominant secretory defect with insulin resistance. It is diagnosed with a fasting blood glucose level of >/- 7.0 mmol/L.

REFERENCES

CHAPTER 1

Alexander, C. "The Coming of Age of the Metabolic Syndrome." *Diabetes Care* 2003; 26(11):3180–3181.

Arbeeny, C., R. Saccheiro, and M. Booker. "The Metabolic Syndrome: From Pathophysiology to Novel Treatment Strategies." *Current Medical Chemistry Immunolgy, Endocrinology & Metabolic Agents* 2001; 1:1–24.

Canadian Diabetes Association. www.diabetes.ca. "What Is Prediabetes?"

Candales-Lopez, A. "Metabolic Syndrome X: A Comprehensive Review of the Pathophysiology and Recommended Therapy." *Journal of Medicine* 2001; 32(5):283–300.

Deedwania, P. "Metabolic Syndrome and Vascular Disease: Is Nature or Nurture Leading the Epidemic of Cardiovascular Disease?" *Circulation* 2004; 109:2–4.

Edleson, Ed. "Get Fit to Fight Metabolic Syndrome." www.medicinenet.com. July 11, 2005.

Ford, E., W. Giles, and W. Dietz. "Prevalence of the Metabolic Syndrome among U.S. Adults: Findings from the Third National Health and Nutrition Examination Survey." *JAMA* 2002; 287(3):356–359.

Harding, Anne. "Stopping Prediabetes in Its Tracks." www.msnbc.com. October 30, 2005.

Hill, J. "What to Do about the Metabolic Syndrome." *Archives of Internal Medicine* 2003; 163:395–397.

Jing, Chen, Rachel Wildman, L. Hamm et al. "Association between Inflammation and Insulin Resistance in U.S. Nondiabetic Adults: Results from the Third National Health and Nutrition Examination Survey." *Diabetes Care* 2004; 27(12):2690–2697.

Laaksonen, D., L. Niskanen, H.M. Lakka et al. "Epidemiology and Treatment of the Metabolic Syndrome." *Annals of Medicine* 2004; 36:332–346.

Lorenzo, C., M. Okoloise, K. Williams et al. "The Metabolic Syndrome as Predictor of Type 2 Diabetes: The San Antonio Heart Study." *Diabetes Care* 2003; 26(11):3153–3159.

Rao, S., P. Disraeli, and T. McGregor. "Impaired Glucose Tolerance and Impaired Fasting Glucose." *American Family Physician* 2004; 69:1961–1968, 1971–1972.

Rigby, Alison. "Insulin Resistance—A Weighty Issue. *Today's Dietitian* 2004; 6(9):46.

Salinas-Aguilar, C., R. Rojas, F. Perez-Gomez et al. "The Metabolic Syndrome: A Concept Hard to Define." *Archives of Medical Research* 2005; 36:223–231.

Schulze, M., and Frank Hu. "Dietary Approaches to Prevent the Metabolic Syndrome." *Diabetes Care* February 2004; 27(2):613–614.

Sutherland, J., B. McKinley, R. Eckel. "The Metabolic Syndrome and Inflammation." *Metabolic Syndrome and Related Disorders* 2004; 2(2):82–104.

Vega, Gloria Lena. "Obesity, the Metabolic Syndrome, and Cardiovascular Disease." *American Heart Journal* 2001; 142:1108–1116.

CHAPTER 2

Challem, Jack. "Paleolithic Nutrition: Your Future Is in Your Dietary Past." www.thenutritionreporter.com.

Clark, Nancy. "Dietary Guidelines: The Link to Longevity."
www.naturalstrength.com. March 2005.

Cordain, L, S.B. Eaton, A. Sebastian, N. Mann et al. "Origins and
Evolution of the Western Diet: Health Implications for the 21st Century."
American Journal of Clinical Nutrition 2005; 81(2):341–354.

Larsen, C.S. "Animal Source Foods and Human Health During Evolution."
Journal of Nutrition 2003; 133(11S-II).

Lindeberg, S. "Paleolithic Diet." *Scandinavian Journal of Nutrition* 2005;
49(2):75–77.

Lindeberg, S., L. Cordain, and S.B. Eaton. "Biological and Clinical
Potential of a Paleolithic Diet." *Journal of Nutritional and Environmental
Medicine* 2003; 13(3):149–160.

Milton, K. "Nutritional Characteristics of Wild Primate Foods: Do the
Diets of Our Closest Living Relatives Have Lessons for Us?" *Nutrition* 1999;
15(6):488–498.

Nestle, M. "Paleolithic Diets: A Skeptical View." *Nutrition Bulletin* 2000;
25(1):43–47.

"What Is the Healthiest Diet for the Human Animal?"
www.naturalhub.com. 2003.

CHAPTER 3

Arita, M., F. Bianchini, J. Aliberti et al. "Stereochemical Assignment, Anti-
inflammatory Properties, and Receptor for the Omega-3 Lipid Mediator
Resolvin E1." *Journal of Experimental Medicine* 2005; 201(5):713–722.

Belury, M.A. "Role of Conjugated Linolenic Acid in the Management of
Type 2 Diabetes: Evidence from Zucker Diabetic Rats and Human Subjects."
American Chemical Society National Meeting, Washington, D.C., August
21, 2000.

Coppack, C. "Pro-inflammatory Cytokines and Adipose Tissue." *Proceedings
of the Nutrition Society* 2001; 60:379–356.

Das, U.N., et al. "Clinical Significance of Essential Fatty Acids." *Nutrition* 1998; 4:337.

Delarue, J., C. Lefoll, C. Corporeau, D. Lucas. "N-3 Chain Polyunsaturated Fatty Acids: A Nutritional Tool to Prevent Insulin Resistance Associated to Type 2 Diabetes and Obesity?" *Reproductive Nutrition Development.* 2004; 44(33):289–299.

Dubnov, G., and E. Berry. "Polyunsaturated Fatty Acids, Insulin Resistance, and Atherosclerosis: Is Inflammation the Connecting Link?" *Metabolic Syndrome and Related Disorders* 2004; 2(2):124–128.

Fan, Y.Y., and R.S. Chapkin. "Importance of Dietary Gamma Linolenic Acid in Human Health and Nutrition." *Journal of Nutrition* 1998; 128:1411–1414.

Fung-Epps, M., J. Williford, Al Wells, and R. Hardy. "Fatty Acid-Induced Insulin Resistance in Adipocytes." *Endocrinology* 1997; 138(10):4338–4345.

Grundy, S.M., N. Abate, and M. Chandalia. "Diet Composition and the Metabolic Syndrome: What Is the Optimal Fat Intake?" *American Journal of Medicine* 2002; 113: Supplement 9B:25S–29S.

Holt, Stephen. "Natural Approaches to Managing Metabolic Syndrome." *Natural Pharmacy* December 2003:10–11.

Horrobin, D., "The Importance of Gamma Linolenic Acid and Prostaglandin E1 in Human Nutrition and Medicine." *Journal of Holistic Medicine* 1981; 3(2):118–136.

Hunnicutt, J.W., R.W. Hardy, J. Williford, and J.M. McDonald. "Saturated Fatty Acid-Induced Insulin Resistance in Rat Adipocytes." *Diabetes* 1994; 43(5):540–545.

Lenhard, J. "The Effect of Fat vs. Carbohydrate on the Etiology of Type 2 Diabetes." www.medscape.com. Sessions of the American Diabetes Association, June 10, 2000.

Louheranta, A.M., A.K. Turpeinen, H.M. Vidgren et al. "A High-Trans Fatty Acid Diet and Insulin Sensitivity in Young Healthy Women." *Metabolism* 1999; 48(7):870–875.

Ludwig, D.S. "Diet and Development of the Insulin Resistance Syndrome." *Asia Pacific Journal of Clinical Nutrition* 2003; 12(S4).

Mann, G.V. "Metabolic Consequences of Dietary Trans Fatty Acids." *Lancet* 1994; 343(8909):1268–1271.

Montori, V., et al. "Fish Oil Supplementation in Type 2 Diabetes." *Diabetes Care* 2000; 23:1407–1415.

Rupp, H., D. Wagner, T. Rupp et al. "Risk Stratification by the EPA+DHA Level and the EPA/AA Ratio." *Herz* 2004; 29:673–685.

Ruxton, C., P. Calder, S. Reed, and M. Simpson. "The Impact of Long-Chain n-3 Polyunsaturated Fatty Acids on Human Health." *Nutrition Research Reviews* 2005; 18:113–129.

"Saturated and Trans Fats, a Risk Factor for Diabetes?" www.nutraingredients.com. June 29, 2005.

Simoncikova, P., S. Wein, D. Gasperikova, J. Ukropec et al. "Comparison of the Extrapancreatic Action of Gamma Linolenic Acid of n-3 PUFAs in the High Fat Diet-Induced Insulin Resistance." *Endocrine Regulations* 2002; 36(4):143–149.

Simopoulos, A.P. "Is Insulin Resistance Influenced by Dietary Linoleic Acid and Trans Fatty Acids?" *Free Radical Biology and Medicine*, 1994; 17(4):367–372.

Sirtori, C., G. Crepaldi, E. Manzato, and M. Mancini. "One-Year Treatment with Ethyl Esters of n-3 Fatty Acids in Patients with Hypertriglceyeridemia and Glucose Intolerance. Reduced triglyceridemia, Total Cholesterol and Increased HDL-C without Glycemic Alterations." *Atherosclerosis* 1998; 137:419–427.

Suresh, Y., and U.N. Das. "Long-Chain Polyunsaturated Fatty Acids and Chemically Induced Diabetes Mellitus: Effect of Omega-3 Fatty Acids." *Nutrition* 2003; 19(3):213–228.

CHAPTER 4

Brand-Miller, J., Hayne S, Petocz P et al. "Low-Glycemic Index Diets in the Management of Diabetes: A Meta-analysis of Randomized Controlled Trials." *Diabetes Care* 2003; 26:2261–2267.

Esmaillzadeh, A., P. Mirmiran, and F. Azizi. "Whole-Grain Consumption and the Metabolic Syndrome: A Favorable Association in Tehranian Adults." *European Journal of Clinical Nutrition* 2005; 59(3):353–362.

Foster-Powell, K., S.H. Holt, and J.C. Brand-Miller. "International Table of Glycemic Index and Glycemic Load Values." *American Journal of Clinical Nutrition* 2002; 5–56.

Harvard School of Public Health. "Carbohydrates: Going with the Whole Grain." www.hsph.harvard.edu. 2005.

Liese, A., A. Roach, K. Sparks et al. "Whole-Grain Intake and Insulin Sensitivity: The Insulin Resistance Atherosclerosis Study." *American Journal of Clinical Nutrition* 2003; 78(5):965–971.

McKeown, N.M., J.B. Meigs, S. Liu et al. "Carbohydrate Nutrition, Insulin Resistance, and the Prevalence of the Metabolic Syndrome in the Framingham Offspring Cohort." *Diabetes Care* 2004; 27(2):538–546.

Mercola, Joseph. "Aspartame: What You Don't Know Can Hurt You." www.mercola.com. 2005.

Reaven, G.M. "Insulin Resistance/Compensatory Hyperinsulinemia, Essential Hypertension, and Cardiovascular Disease." *Journal of Clinical Endocrinology and Metabolism* 2003; 88:2399–2403.

Salmeron, J., J.E. Manson, M.F. Stampfer et al. "Dietary Fiber, Glycemic Load, and Risk of Non-insulin Dependent Diabetes Mellitus in Women." JAMA 1997; 277)6):472–476.

Schulze, M., and Frank Hu. "Dietary Approaches to Prevent Metabolic Syndrome." *Diabetes Care* 2004; 27:613–614.

Schulze, M.B., S. Liu, E.B. Rimm, J.E. Manson et al. "Glycemic Index, Glycemic Load, and Dietary Fiber Intake and Incidence of Type 2 Diabetes in Younger and Middle-Age Women." *American Journal of Clinical Nutrition* 2004; 80:348–356.

Warner, Jennifer. "High Fiber Cereal May Ward off Diabetes." www.mywebmd.com. June 18, 2004.

www.xylitol.org.

CHAPTER 5

Astrup, A. "The Satiating Power of Protein: A Key to Obesity Prevention?" *American Journal of Clinical Nutrition* 2005; 82:1–2.

Ceriello, A. "The Possible Role of Postprandial Hyperglycemia in the Pathogenesis of Diabetic Complications." *Diabetologia* 2003; 46(Supplement):M9–16.

Charlton, M., and K.S. Nair. "Protein Metabolism in Insulin-Dependent Diabetes Mellitus." *Journal of Nutrition* 1998; 128(Supplement):S323–327.

Frid, A., M. Nilsson, J. Holst, and I. Bjorck. "Effect of Whey on Blood Glucose and Insulin Responses to Composite Breakfast and Lunch Meals in Type 2 Diabetic Subjects." *American Journal of Clinical Nutrition* 2005; 82:69–75.

Gannon, M.C., F.Q. Nutall, B.J. Neil, and S.A. Westphal. "The Insulin and Glucose Responses to Meals of Glucose Plus Various Proteins in Type II Diabetic Subjects." *Metabolism* 1988; 37:1081–1088.

Manders, R., A. Wagenmakers, R. Koopman et al. "Co-ingestion of a Protein Hydrolysate and Amino Acid Mixture with Carbohydrate Improves Plasma Glucose Disposal in Patients with Type 2 Diabetes." *American Journal of Clinical Nutrition* 2005; 82:76–83.

Sachiko, T., B. Howard, E. Prewitt, V. Bovee et al. "Dietary Protein and Weight Reduction." *Circulation* 2001; 104:1869.

Whey Protein Institute. "Benefits of Whey Protein." www.wheyoflife.org 2005.

CHAPTER 6

Aude, Y., P. Mego, and J. Mehta. "Metabolic Syndrome: Dietary Interventions." *Current Opinion in Cardiology* 2004; 19:473–479.

Birmingham, C.L., J.L. Muller, A. Palepu et al. "The Cost of Obesity in Canada." *CMAJ* 1999; 160(4):483–488. www.cmaj.ca/cgi/reprint/160/4/483.

Bjorntorp, P., and R. Rosmond. "Obesity and Cortisol." *Nutrition* 2000; 16:924–936.

Blackburn, G., and L. Bevis. "The Obesity Epidemic: Prevention and Treatment of the Metabolic Syndrome." www.medscape.com. 2003.

Brotman, D., and J. Girod. "The Metabolic Syndrome: A Tug-of-War with No Winner." *Cleveland Clinical Journal of Medicine* 2002; 69(12):990–994.

Katzmarzyk, P. "The Canadian Obesity Epidemic." CMAJ 2002; 166(8). www.cmaj.ca/cgi/content/full/.

National Institute of Health. "Clinical Guidelines on the Identification, Evaluation, and Treatment of Overweight and Obesity in Adults." Bethesda: National Institute of Health, 1998. www.nhlbi.nih.gov/guidelines/obesity/ob_home.htm.

Raine, K. "Overweight and Obesity in Canada: A Population Health Perspective." Calgary: Centre for Health Promotion Studies, University of Alberta, August 2004.

Ramos, E., Y. Xu, I. Romanova et al. "Is Obesity an Inflammatory Disease?" *Surgery* 2003; 134:329–335.

Riccardi, G., and A.A. Rivellese. "Dietary Treatment of the Metabolic Syndrome—the Optimal Diet." *British Journal of Nutrition* 2000; 83(Supplement 1):S143–S148.

U.S. Department of Health and Human Services. "The Surgeon General's Call to Action to Prevent and Decrease Overweight and Obesity." Rockville: U.S. Department of Health and Human Services, Public Health Service, Office of the Surgeon General, 2001. www.surgeongeneral.gov/sgoffice.htm.

World Health Organization. *Obesity: Preventing and Managing the Global Epidemic*. Geneva: The World Health Organization, 2000. Technical Report Series no. 894.

CHAPTER 7

AHA Scientific Statement: Diabetes and Cardiovascular Disease, #71-0175. *Circulation* 1999; 100:1134–1146.

Dominiczak, M. "Obesity, Glucose Intolerance and Diabetes and Their Links to Cardiovascular Disease: Implications for Laboratory Medicine." *Clinical Chemistry and Laboratory Medicine* 2003; 41(9):1266–1278.

Gannon, M.C., and F.Q. Nuttall. "Effect of a High-Protein, Low-Carbohydrate Diet on Blood Glucose Control in People with Type 2 Diabetes." *Diabetes* 2004; 53(9):2375–2382.

Gross, L.S., et al. "Increased Consumption of Refined Carbohydrates and the Epidemic of Type 2 Diabetes in the United States: An Ecologic Assessment." *American Journal of Clinical Nutrition* 2004; 79(5):774–779.

Hanson, R., G. Imperatore, P. Bennett, and W. Knowler. "Components of the Metabolic Syndrome and Incidence of Type 2 Diabetes." *Diabetes* 2002; 51(10):3120–3127.

Hart, C., and M. Grossman. *The Insulin Resistance Diet*. Chicago, IL: Contemporary Books, 2001.

Jeejeebhoy, K. "The Nutrition Factor: Insulin Resistance a Big Contributor to Health Cost." *The Medical Post* April 13, 2000; 36(14):1-2.

Lautt, W. "A Proposed New Paradigm for Insulin Resistance." *Metabolic Syndrome and Related Disorders* 2003; 1(4):261–270.

Meckling, K.A., C. O'Sullivan, and D. Saari. "Comparison of a Low-Fat Diet to a Low-Carbohydrate Diet on Weight Loss, Body Composition and Risk Factors for Diabetes and Cardiovascular Disease in Free-Living, Overweight Men and Women. *Journal of Clinical Endocrinology and Metabolism* 2004; 89(6):2717–2723.

Murray, M., and M. Lyon. *How to Prevent and Treat Diabetes with Natural Medicine*. New York, NY: Riverhead Books, 2003.

Parillo, M., and G. Riccardi. "Diet Composition and the Risk of Type 2 Diabetes: Epidemiological and Clinical Evidence." *British Journal of Nutrition* 2004; 92(1):7–19.

PR Newswire. "New European Study Exmaines the Role of Insulin Resistance in Predicting Cardiovascular Disease." September 3, 2004.

Segal, P., and P. Zimmet. "1st International Congress on Prediabetes and the Metabolic Syndrome, April 13–16, 2005." *Medscape Diabetes & Endocrinology* 2005; 7(2). www.medscape.com/viewrticle/506474.

Voss, L., J. Kirkby, B. Metcalf et al. "Preventable Factors in Childhood That Lead to Insulin Resistance, Diabetes Mellitus and the Metabolic Syndrome: The Earlybird Diabetes Study 1." *Journal of Pediatric Endocrinology & Metabolism* 2003; 16:1211–1224.

Zimmett, P. "The Global Scope of Diabetes and Obesity—An Epidemic in Progress: Paradise Lost." Presented at the 60th Scientific Sessions of the American Diabetes Association, San Antonio, Texas, June 10, 2000.

CHAPTER 8

Aljada, Ahmad. "Endothelium, Inflammation, and Diabetes." *Metabolic Syndrome and Related Disorders* 2003; 1(1):3–21.

Barzilay, J., and E. Freedland. "Inflammation and Its Relationship to Insulin Resistance, Type 2 Diabetes Mellitus, and Endothelial Dysfunction." *Metabolic Syndrome and Related Disorders* 2003; 1(1):55–67.

Chilton, F. *The Inflammation Nation*. New York, NY: Simon & Schuster, 2005.

Dandona, P., A. Aljada, and A. Chaudhuri. "A Novel View of Metabolic Syndrome." *Metabolic Syndrome and Related Disorders* 2004; 2(1):2–8.

Dandona, P., A. Aljada, A. O'Donnell et al. "Insulin Is an Anti-inflammatory and Anti-atherosclerotic Hormone." *Metabolic Syndrome and Related Disorders* 2004; 2(2):137–142.

Lee, Y., and R. Pratley. "The Evolving Role of Inflammation in Obesity and the Metabolic Syndrome." *Current Diabetes Reports* 2005; 5(1):70–75.

Loebner, K., and M. Fouchtenbusch. "Inflammation and Diabetes." *MMW Fortschr Medicine* 2004; 146(35–36):32–33, 35–36.

Ridker, P., J. Buring, N. Cook, and N. Rifai. "C-Reactive Protein, the Metabolic Syndrome, and Risk of Incident Cardiovascular Events." *Circulation* 2003; 107:391–397.

Savage, D., K. Petersen, and G. Shulman. "Mechanisms of Insulin Resistance in Humans as Possible Links with Inflammation." *Hypertension* 2005; 45(5):828–833.

Schulze, M., K. Hoffmann, J. Manson et al. "Dietary Pattern, Inflammation and Incidence of Type 2 Diabetes in Women." *American Journal of Clinical Nutrition* 2005; 82(3):675–684.

Sears, B., and S. Bell. "The Zone Diet: An Anti-Inflammatory, Low Glycemic-Load Diet." *Metabolic Syndrome and Related Disorders* 2004; 2(1):24–38.

Sjoholm, A., and M. Nystrol. "Endothelial Inflammation in Insulin Resistance." *Lancet* 2005; 365:610–612.

Sutherland, J., B. McKinley, and R. Eckel. "The Metabolic Syndrome and Inflammation." *Metabolic Syndrome and Related Disorders* 2004; 2(2):82–104.

Theuma, P. "Inflammation, Insulin Resistance, and Atherosclerosis." *Metabolic Syndrome and Related Disorders* 2004; 2(2):105–113.

Trayhurn, P., and I.S. Wood. "Adipokines: Inflammation and the Pleiotropic Role of White Adipose Tissue." *British Journal of Nutrition* 2005; 92(3):347–355.

Ziegler, D. "Type 2 Diabetes as an Inflammatory Cardiovascular Disorder." *Current Molecular Medicine* 2005; 5(3):309–322.

CHAPTER 9

Alexander, C.M., P.B. Landsman, S.M. Teutsch, and S.M. Haffner. "Third National Health and Nutrition Examination Survey 9 NHANES III). National Cholesterol Education Program (NCEP). NCEP-Defined Metabolic Syndrome, Diabetes, and Prevalence of Coronary Heart Disease among NHANES III Participants Age 50 Years and Older." *Diabetes* 2003; 52:1210–1241.

Berger, D., and A. Harmel. "Clinical Implications of the Metabolic Syndrome." www.medscape.com/viewarticle/462881.

"Expert Panel on Detection, Evaluation and Treatment of High Blood Cholesterol in Adults: Executive Summary of the Third Report of the National Cholesterol Education Program (NCEP)." JAMA 2001; 285:2486–2497.

Ginsberg, H.N. "Insulin Resistance and Cardiovascular Disease." *Journal of Clinical Investigation* 2000; 106-453–458.

Grundy, S.M. "Hypertriglyceridemia, Insulin Resistance, and the Metabolic Syndrome." *American Journal of Cardiology* 1999; 83:25F–29F.

Isomaa, B., K. Lahti, P. Almgren, M. Nissen, T. Tuomi et al. "Cardiovascular Morbidity and Mortality Associated with the Metabolic Syndrome." *Diabetes Care* 2001; 24(4):683–689.

Lakka, H.M., D.E. Laaksonen, T.A. Lakka et al. "The Metabolic Syndrome and Total and Cardiovascular Disease Mortality in Middle-Aged Men." *JAMA* 2002; 288:2709–2716.

Leiter, L., D. Abbott, N. Campbell et al. "Recommendations on Obesity and Weight Loss." *CMAJ* 1999; 160(9 Supplement):S7–S12.

Reaven, G.M. "Insulin Resistance/Compensatory Hyperinsulinemia, Essential Hypertension, and Cardiovascular Disease." *Journal of Clinical Endocrinology and Metabolism* 2003; 88:2399–2403.

Vitaliano, P., J. Scanlan, J. Zhang et al. "A Path Model of Chronic Stress, the Metabolic Syndrome, and Coronary Heart Disease." *Psychosomatic Medicine* 2002; 64:418–435.

Weber, M. "Hypertension, the Metabolic Syndrome, and the Risk of Developing Diabetes: Is It Time to Change the Guidelines?" *Journal of Clinical Hypertension* 2004; 6(8):425–427, 460.

Wilson, P., and S. Grundy. "The Metabolic Syndrome: A Practical Guide to Origins and Treatment: Part II." *Circulation* 2003; 108:1537–1540.

CHAPTER 10

Anderson, A. "How to Implement Dietary Changes to Prevent the Development of Metabolic Syndrome." *British Journal of Nutrition* 2000; 83(Supplement 1):S165–S168.

Aude, Y., P. Mego, and J. Mehta. "Metabolic Syndrome: Dietary Interventions." *Current Opinion in Cardiology* 2004; 19:473–479.

Health Canada. *Canada's Food Guide to Healthy Eating.* 1992.

Murray, M., and M. Lyon. *How to Prevent and Treat Diabetes with Natural Medicine.* New York, NY: Riverhead Books, 2003.

Nestel, P. "Nutritional Aspects in the Causation and Management of the Metabolic Syndrome." *Endocrinology Metababolism Clin N Am* 2004; 33:483–492.

Sears, B., and S. Bell. "The Zone Diet: An Anti-Inflammatory, Low Glycemic-Load Diet." *Metabolic Syndrome and Related Disorders* 2004; 2(1):24–38.

Stone, N. "Focus on Lifestyle Change and the Metabolic Syndrome." *Endocrinology and Metabolism Clinics of North America* 2004; 33:493–508.

Tapsell, L. "Diet and Metabolic Syndrome: Where Does Resistant Starch Fit in?" *Journal of AOAC International* 2004; 87(3):756–760.

U.S. Department of Agriculture and U.S. Department of Health and Human Services. *Food Guide Pyramid.* 1992.

U.S. Department of Agriculture and U.S. Department of Health and Human Services, *My Pyramid,* 2005.

Wein, M.A., J.M. Sabate, D.N. Ikle, S.E. Cole, and F.R. Kandeel. "Almonds vs. Complex Carbohydrates in a Weight-Reduction Program." *International Journal of Obesity* 2003; 27:1365–1372.

CHAPTER 11

Abuissa, H., D.S. Bel, and J.H. O'Keefe. "Strategies to Prevent Type 2 Diabetes." *Current Medical Research and Opinion* 2005; 21(7):1107–1114.

Annania, F.A., S. Parekh, and A. Shaukat. "The Diabetes Prevention Program and the Metabolic Syndrome." *Annals of Internal Medicine* 2005; 143(7):545.

Biolo, G., B. Ciocchi, M. Stulle et al. "Metabolic Consequences of Physical Inactivity." *Journal of Renal Nutrition* 2005; 15(1):49–53.

Deen, D. "Metabolic Syndrome: Time for Action." *American Family Physician* 2004; 69:2875–2882, 2884–2888.

Fowler, S.B., M. Moussouttas, and B. Mancini. "Metabolic Syndrome: Contributing Factors and Treatment Strategies." *Journal of Neuroscience Nursing* 2005; 37(4):220–223.

Hill, A., J. Buckley, K. Murphy, D. Saint et al. "Combined Effects of Omega-3 Supplementation and Regular Exercise on Body Composition and Cardiovascular Risk Factors." *Asia Pacific Journal of Clinical Nutrition* 2005; 14(Supplement):S57.

Katzmarzyk, P.T., T.S. Church, I. Janssen, R. Ross, and S.N. Blair. "Metabolic Syndrome, Obesity, and Mortality: Impact of Cardiorespiratory Fitness." *Diabetes Care* 2005; 28(2):391–397.

Kousar, R., C. Burns, and P. Lewandowski. "Changes to Diet and Physical Activity Have the Potential to Treat the Metabolic Syndrome in Female Pakistani Immigrants." *Asia Pacific Journal of Clinical Nutrition* 2005; 14(Supplement):S50.

Kukkonen-Harjula, K.T., P.T. Borg, A.M. Nenone, and M.G. Fogelholm. "Effects of a Weight Maintenance Program with or without Exercise on the Metabolic Syndrome: A Randomized Trial in Obese Men." *Preventitive Medicine* 2005; 41(3–4):784–790.

Petersen, A.M., and B.K. Pedersen. "The Anti-inflammatory Effect of Exercise." *Journal of Applied Physiology* 2005; 98(4):1154–1162.

Pitsavos, C., D.B. Panagiotakos, C. Chrysohoou, S. Kavouras, and C. Stefanadis. "The Associations between Physical Activity, Inflammation, and Coagulation Markers in People with Metabolic Syndrome: The ATTICA Study." *European Journal of Cardiovascular Preventitive Rehabilitation* 2005; 12(2):151–158.

Volek, J.S., J.L. Vanheest, and C.E. Forsythe. "Diet and Exercise for Weight Loss: A Review of Current Issues." *Sports Medicine* 2005; 35(1):1–9.

Warner, J., and B. Nazario. "Exercise May Reduce Metabolic Syndrome Risks." www.my.webmd.com/content/Article/97/104009.htm.

CHAPTER 12

Al Shamsi, M.S., A. Amin, and E. Adeghate. "Beneficial Effect of Vitamin E on the Metabolic Parameters of Diabetic Rats." *Mollecular and Cellular Biochemistry* 2004; 261(1):35–42.

Althuis, Jordan N.E., E.A. Ludington, and J.T. Wittes. "Glucose and Insulin Responses to Dietary Chromium Supplements: A Meta-analysis." *American Journal of Clinical Nutrition* 2002; 76:148–155.

Anderson, R.A. "Effects of Chromium on Body Composition and Weight Loss." *Nutrition Reviews* 1998; 56:266–270.

Anderson, R.A. "Chromium in the Prevention and Control of Diabetes." *Diabetes and Metabolism* 2000; 26(1):22–27.

Barbagello, M., et al. "Role of Magnesium in Insulin Action, Diabetes and Cardio-Metabolic Syndrome X." *Mollecular Aspects of Medicine* 2003; 24(1–3):39–52.

Bitar, M.S., et al. "Alpha Lipoic Acid Mitigates Insulin Resistance in Got-Kakizaki Rats." *Hormone and Metabolic Research* 2004; 36(8):542–549.

Boozer, C.N., J.A. Nasser, S.B. Heymsfield et al. "An Herbal Supplement Containing Ma Huang-Guarana for Weight Loss: A Randomized, Double-Blind Trial." *International Journal of Obesity and Related Metabolic Disorder* 2001; 25(3):316–324.

Chausmer, A.B. "Zinc, Insulin and Diabetes." *Journal of the American College of Nutrition* 1998; 17(2):109–115.

Cheng, N., et al. "Hypoglycemic Effects of Cinnamon, Heshouwu and Mushroom Extracts in Type 2 Diabetes Mellitus." *FASEB Journal* 2002; 16(4):A647.

Chew, G.T., and G.F. Watts. "Coenzyme Q10 and Diabetic Endotheliopathy: Oxidative Stress and the Recoupling Hypothesis." *Quarterly Journal of Medicine* 2004; 97(8):537–548.

Crawford, V., R. Scheckenback, and H.G. Preuss. "Effects of Niacin-Bound Chromium Supplementation on Body Composition in Overweight African-American Women." *Diabetes Obesity and Metabolism* 1999; 1:331–337.

DeValk, H.W. "Magnesium in Diabetes Mellitus." *Netherlands Journal of Medicine* 1999; 54(4):139–146.

Guerrero-Romero, F., et al. "Oral Magnesium Supplementation Improves Insulin Sensitivity in Nondiabetic Subjects with Insulin Resistance: A Double-Blind, Placebo-Controlled Randomized Trial." *Diabetes and Metabolism* 2004; 30(3):253–258.

Halliwell, B. "Vitamin E and the Treatment and Prevention of Diabetes: A Case for a Controlled Clinical Trial." *Singapore Medical Journal* 2002; 43(9):479–484.

Hodgson, J.M., et al. "Coenzyme Q10 Improves Blood Pressure and Glycemic Control: A Controlled Trial in Subjects with Type 2 Diabetes." *European Journal of Clinical Nutrition* 2002; 56(11):1137–1142.

Khan, A., et al. "Cinnamon Improves Glucose and Lipids of People with Type 2 Diabetes." *Diabetes Care* 2003; 26(12):3215–3218.

Khosh, F. "A Natural Approach to Diabetes." *The Townsend Letter for Doctors and Patients* 2005.

Kiefer, D., and T. Pantuso. "Panax Ginseng." *Complementary and Alternative Medicine* 2003; 68:1539–1542.

Manning, P.J., et al. "Effect of High-Dose Vitamin E on Insulin Resistance and Associated Parameters in Overweight Subjects." *Diabetes Care* 2004; 27(9):2166–2171.

Medicine Net. "Weight Loss: Over-the Counter and Herbal Remedies for Weight Loss." www.medicinenet.com.

Meyers, C., and M. Kashyap. "Management of the Metabolic Syndrome— Nicotinic Acid." *Endocrinology and Metabolism Clinics of North America* 2004; 33:557–575.

Miranda, E.R., and C.S. Dey. "Effect of Chromium and Zinc on Insulin Signaling in Skeletal Muscle Cells." *Biological Trace Element Research* 2004; 101(1):19–36.

Montonen, J., et al. "Dietary Antioxidant Intake and Risk of Type 2 Diabetes." *Diabetes Care* 2004; 27(2):362–366.

Nettleton, J., and R. Katz. "n-3 Long-Chain Polyunsaturated Fatty Acids in Type 2 Diabetes." *Journal of the American Dietetic Association* 2005; 105(93):428–440.

Noakes, M., P. Foster, J. Keogh, and P. Clifton. "Meal Replacements Are as Effective as Structured Weight-Loss Diets for Treating Obesity in Adults with Features of Metabolic Syndrome." *Journal of Nutrition* 2004; 134:1894–1899.

PDR Health. "Glucomannan." www.pdrhealth.com/drug_info.

Pittas, A. "Nutrition Interventions for Prevention of Type 2 Diabetes and the Metabolic Syndrome." *Nutrition Clinical Care* 2003; 6:79–88.

Porchezhian, E., and R.M. Dobriyal. "An Overview on the Advances of Gymnema sylvestre: Chemistry, Pharmacology and Patents." *Pharmazie* 2003; 58(1):5–12.

Preuss, H.G., D. Bagchi, M. Bagchi et al. "Effects of a Natural Extract of Hydroxycitric Acid and a Combination of HCA-SX Plus Niacin-Bound Chromium and Gymnema sylvestre Extract on Weight Loss." *Diabetes, Obesity & Metabolism* 2004; 6:171–180.

Rabinovitz, H., et al. "Effect of Chromium Supplementation on Blood Glucose and Lipid Levels in Type 2 Diabetes Mellitus Elderly Patients." *International Journal of Vitamin and Nutrition Research.* 2004; 3:178–182.

Ramos, R.R., J.L.F. Senz, and F.J.A. Aguilar. "Extract of *Garcinia cambogia* in Controlling Obesity." *Investigacin Medica Internacional* 1995; 22:97–101.

Rodriguez-Moran, M., and F. Guerrero-Romero. "Oral Magnesium Supplementation Improves Insulin Sensitivity and Metabolic Control in Type 2 Diabetic Subjects: A Randomized Double-Blind Controlled Trial." *Diabetes Care* 2003; 26(4):1147–1152.

Ryan, G.J., et al. "Chromium as Adjunctive Treatment for Type 2 Diabetes." *Annals of Pharmacotherapy* 2003; 37(6):876–885.

Sakurai, H. "A New Concept: The Use of Vanadium Complexes in the Treatment of Diabetes Mellitus." *Chemical Record* 2002; 2(4):237–248.

Saper, R., D. Eisenberg, and R. Phillips. "Common Dietary Supplements for Weight Loss." *American Family Physician* 2004; 70(9):1731–1738.

Song, Y., et al. "Dietary Magnesium Intake in Relation to Plasma Insulin Levels and Risk of Type 2 Diabetes in Women." *Diabetes Care* 2004; 27(1):59–65.

Thom, E. "Hydroxycitrate (HCA) in the Treatment of Obesity." *International Journal of Obesity* 1996; 20:75.

Tsuneki, H., et al. "Effects of Green Tea on Blood Glucose Levels and Serum Proteomic Patterns in Diabetic Mice and on Glucose Metabolism in Healthy Humans." BMC *Clinical Pharmacology* 2004; 4(1):18.

Yeh, G.Y., et al. "Systematic Review of Herbs and Dietary Supplements for Glycemic Control in Diabetes." *Diabetes Care* 2003; 26(4):1277–1294.

INDEX